Health Care Finance

Basic Tools for Nonfinancial Managers

Second Edition

Judith J. Baker, PhD, CPA
Executive Director
Resource Group, Ltd.
Dallas, Texas

R.W. Baker, JD
Managing Partner
Resource Group, Ltd.
Dallas, Texas

JONES AND BARTLETT PUBLISHERS
Sudbury, Massachusetts
BOSTON   TORONTO   LONDON   SINGAPORE

World Headquarters

Jones and Bartlett Publishers
40 Tall Pine Drive
Sudbury, MA 01776
978-443-5000
info@jbpub.com
www.jbpub.com

Jones and Bartlett Publishers
Canada
6339 Ormindale Way
Mississauga, ON L5V 1J2
Canada

Jones and Bartlett Publishers
International
Barb House, Barb Mews
London W6 7PA
United Kingdom

Jones and Bartlett's books and products are available through most bookstores and online booksellers. To contact Jones and Bartlett Publishers directly, call 800-832-0034, fax 978-443-8000, or visit our website at www.jbpub.com.

ISBN-13: 978-0-7637-2660-7
ISBN-10: 0-7637-2660-5

LIBRARY OF CONGRESS CATALOGING-IN-PUBLICATION DATA
Baker, Judith J.
    Health care finance : basic tools for nonfinancial managers /
Judith Baker, R.W. Baker.— 2nd ed.
        p. cm.
    Includes bibliographical references and index.
    ISBN 0-7637-2660-5 (pbk.)
    1. Health facilities—Finance—Case studies. 2. Health facilities—Accounting—Case studies.
    [DNLM: 1. Financial Management—United States. 2. Delivery of Health Care—
    economics—United States. 3. Health Facilities—economics—United States. 4. Health
    Facilities—organization & administration—United States. W 74 AA1 B167h 2006]
    I. Baker, R. W.   II. Title.
    RA971.3.B353 2006
    362.1'068'1—dc22

                        2005023424

6048

PRODUCTION CREDITS
Publisher: Michael Brown
Associate Editor: Kylah Goodfellow McNeill
Production Director: Amy Rose
Associate Production Editor: Kate Hennessy
Associate Marketing Manager: Marissa Hederson
Manufacturing Buyer: Therese Connell
Composition: Pageworks
Cover Design: Kristin E. Ohlin
Printing and Binding: Malloy, Inc.
Cover Printing: Malloy, Inc.

Printed in the United States of America
13 12 11 10 09   10 9 8 7 6 5

Table of Contents

Preface

Our world of work is divided into three parts: the health care consultant, the instructor, and the writer. Over the years, we have taught managers in seminars, in academic settings, and in corporate conference rooms. Most of the managers were mid-career adults, working in all types of health care disciplines. We taught them, and they taught us. One of the things they taught us was this: a nonfinancial manager pushed into dealing with the world of finance often feels a dislocation and a change of perspective, and that experience can be both difficult and exciting. We have listened to their questions and concerns as these managers grapple with this new world. This book is the result of their experiences, and ours.

The book is designed for use by a manager (or future manager) who does not have an educational background in financial management. It has long been our philosophy that if you can truly understand how a thing works—whatever it is—then you own it. This book is created around that philosophy. In other words, we intend to make financial management transparent by showing how it works and how a manager can use it.

USING THE BOOK

Users will find examples and exercises covering many types of health care settings and providers included. The case study of Metropolis Hospital System is woven throughout the book. Three mini-case studies are provided to give an even broader view of the subjects covered. "Progress Notes" set out learning objectives at the beginning of each chapter. An "Information Checkpoint" segment at the end of each chapter tells the user three things: information needed, where this information can be obtained, and how this information can be used. A "Key Terms" section follows the "Information Checkpoint." Each of these features displays its own quick-reference icon.

Easy access to the Web site is also shown in Appendix B, "Web-Based Learning Tools." For users who prefer a calculator, Appendix B provides guidance on where to obtain information on using a business analyst calculator. And for those users who choose neither a computer nor a calculator, instructions are set out so problems can also be worked by hand, with paper and pencil.

Acknowledgments

The book originated during the course of our activity-based costing seminars for Irwin Professional Seminars, when class members kept inserting finance questions into the sessions. The original concept for the book was clarified when Cleo Boulter, then Associate Professor at the University of Texas at Houston Center on Aging, recruited us to teach intensive finance sessions to her mid-career students, an arrangement that continued over a period of years. The needs of these students and their reaction to the material provided the core of the book's first edition content.

Special thanks go to John Brocketti, Chief Financial Office, SUMA Health System, Akron, Ohio, to Christine Pierce, Partner, The Resource Group, Cleveland, Ohio, and to numerous instructors for their information and suggestions concerning the second edition.

Our continued gratitude goes to Craig Sheagren, Senior Vice President/CFO, McDonough District Hospital, Macomb, Illinois, and Nancy M. Borkowski, PhD, Professor, Dept of Professional Management/Health Management, St. Thomas University, Miami, Florida for their encouragement, information, suggestions and assistance with the original concept of the book.

Dr. Frank Welsh, Cincinnati, Ohio, contributed a new case study about managed care contracts to this second edition. Many others also contributed suggestions, recommendations, and information to help shape and refine the initial concept. We continue to acknowledge these individuals, listed below, including their original affiliations:

Ian G. Worden, CPA, Regional Vice President of Finance/CFO, PeaceHealth, Eugene, Oregon

Carol A. Robinson, Medical Records Director, Titus Regional Medical Center, Mt. Pleasant, Texas

John Congelli, Vice President of Finance, Genesee Memorial Hospital, Batavia, New York

Charles A. Keil, Cost Accountant, Genesee Memorial Hospital, Batavia, New York

George O. Kimbro, CPA, CFO, Hunt Memorial Hospital District, Greenville, Texas

Bob Gault, Laboratory Director, Hunt Memorial Hospital District, Greenville, Texas

Ted J. Stuart, Jr. MD, MBA, Northwest Family Physicians, Glendale, Arizona

Mark Potter, EMS Director, Hopkins County Memorial Hospital, Sulphur Springs, Texas

and

Leonard H. Friedman, PhD, Assistant Professor, Coordinator, Health Care Administration Program, Oregon State University, Corvallis, Oregon

Patricia Chiverton, EdD, RN, Dean, University of Rochester School of Nursing, Rochester, New York

Donna M. Tortoretti, RNC, Chief Operating Officer, Community Nursing Center, University of Rochester School of Nursing, Rochester, New York

Billie Ann Brotman, PhD, Professor of Finance, Dept of Economics and Finance, Kennesaw State University, Kennesaw, Georgia

PART I

Health Care Finance Overview

CHAPTER 1

Introduction to Health Care Finance

PROGRESS NOTES

After completing this chapter you should be able to

1. Discuss the three viewpoints of managers in organizations.
2. Identify the four elements of financial management.
3. Understand the differences between the two types of accounting.
4. Identify the types of organizations.
5. Understand the composition and purpose of an organization chart.

THE HISTORY

Financial management has a long and distinguished history. Consider, for example, that Socrates wrote about the universal function of management in human endeavors in 400 B.C. and that Plato developed the concept of specialization for efficiency in 350 B.C. Evidence of sophisticated financial management exists for much earlier times: the Chinese produced a planning and control system in 1100 B.C., a minimum-wage system was developed by Hammurabi in 1800 B.C., and the Egyptians and Sumerians developed planning and record-keeping systems in 4000 B.C.[1]

Many managers in early history discovered and rediscovered managerial principles while attempting to reach their goals. Because the idea of management thought as a discipline had not yet evolved, they formulated principles of management because certain goals had to be accomplished. As management thought became codified over time, however, the building of techniques for management became more organized. Management as a discipline for educational purposes began in the United States in 1881. On that date, Joseph Wharton created the Wharton School, offering college courses in business management at the University of Pennsylvania. It was the only such school until 1898, when the Universities of Chicago and California established their business schools. Thirteen years later, in 1911, 30 such schools were in operation in the United States.[2]

Over the long span of history, managers have all sought how to make organizations work more effectively. Financial management is a vital part of organizational effectiveness.

This book's goal is to provide the keys to unlock the secrets of financial management for nonfinancial managers.

THE CONCEPT

A Method of Getting Money in and out of the Business

One of our colleagues, a nurse, talks about the area of health care finance as "a method of getting money in and out of the business." It is not a bad description. As we shall see, revenues represent inflow and expenses represent outflow. Thus, "getting money in" represents the inflow (revenues), whereas "getting money out" (expenses) represents the outflow. The successful manager, through planning, organizing, controlling, and decision making, is able to adjust the inflow and outflow to achieve the most beneficial outcome for the organization.

HOW DOES FINANCE WORK IN THE HEALTH CARE BUSINESS?

The purpose of this book is to show how the various elements of finance fit together: in other words, how finance works in the health care business. The real key to understanding finance is understanding the various pieces and their relationship to each other. If you, the manager, truly see how the elements work, then they are yours. They become your tools to achieve management success.

The health care industry is a service industry. It is not in the business of manufacturing, say, widgets. Instead, its essential business is the delivery of health care services. It may have inventories of medical supplies and drugs, but those inventories are necessary to service delivery, not to manufacturing functions. Because the business of health care is service, the explanations and illustrations within this book focus on the practice of financial management in the service industries.

VIEWPOINTS

The managers within a health care organization will generally have one of three views: (1) financial, (2) process, or (3) clinical. The way they manage will be influenced by which view they hold.

1. *The financial view.* These managers generally work with finance on a daily basis. The reporting function is part of their responsibility. They usually perform much of the strategic planning for the organization.
2. *The process view.* These managers generally work with the system of the organization. They may be responsible for data accumulation. They are often affiliated with the information system hierarchy in the organization.
3. *The clinical view.* These managers generally are responsible for service delivery. They have direct interaction with the patients and are responsible for clinical outcomes of the organization.

Managers must, of necessity, interact with one another. Thus, managers holding different views will be required to work together. Their concerns will intersect to some degree, as illustrated by Figure 1-1. The nonfinancial manager who understands health care finance will be able to interpret and negotiate successfully such interactions between and among viewpoints.

In summary, financial management is a discipline with a long and respected history. Health care service delivery is a business, and the concept of financial management assists in balancing the inflows and outflows that are a part of the business.

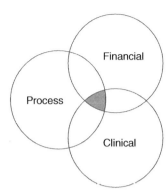

Figure 1–1 Three Views of Management within an Organization.

WHY MANAGE?

Business does not run itself. It requires a variety of management activities in order to operate properly.

THE ELEMENTS OF FINANCIAL MANAGEMENT

There are four recognized elements of financial management: (1) planning, (2) controlling, (3) organizing and directing, and (4) decision making. The four divisions are based on the purpose of each task. Some authorities stress only three elements (planning, controlling, and decision making) and consider organizing and directing as a part of the controlling element. This text recognizes organizing and directing as a separate element of financial management, primarily because such a large proportion of managers' time is taken up with performing these duties.

1. *Planning.* The financial manager identifies the steps that must be taken to accomplish the organization's objectives. Thus, the purpose is to identify objectives and then to identify the steps required for accomplishing these objectives.

2. *Controlling.* The financial manager makes sure that each area of the organization is following the plans that have been established. One way to do this is to study current reports and compare them with reports from earlier periods. This comparison often shows where the organization may need attention because that area is not effective. The reports that the manager uses for this purpose are often called *feedback.* The purpose of controlling is to ensure that plans are being followed.

3. *Organizing and directing.* When organizing, the financial manager decides how to use the resources of the organization to most effectively carry out the plans that have been established. When directing, the manager works on a day-to-day basis to keep the results of the organizing running efficiently. The purpose is to ensure effective resource use and provide daily supervision.

4. *Decision making.* The financial manager makes choices among available alternatives. Decision making actually occurs parallel to planning, organizing, and controlling. All types of decision making rely on information, and the primary tasks are analysis and evaluation. Thus, the purpose is to make informed choices.

THE ORGANIZATION'S STRUCTURE

The structure of an organization is an important factor in management.

Organization Types

Organizations fall into one of two basic types: profit oriented or nonprofit oriented.

In the United States, these designations follow the taxable status of the organizations. The profit-oriented entities, also known as *proprietary organizations*, are responsible for paying income taxes. Proprietary subgroups include individuals, partnerships, and corporations. The nonprofit organizations do not pay income taxes.

There are two subgroups of nonprofit entities: voluntary and government. Voluntary nonprofits have sought tax-exempt status. In general, voluntary nonprofits are associated with churches, private schools, or foundations. Government nonprofits, on the other hand, do not pay taxes because they are government entities. Government nonprofits can be (1) federal, (2) state, (3) county, (4) city, (5) a combination of city and county, (6) a hospital taxing district (with the power to raise revenues through taxes), or (7) a state university (perhaps with a teaching hospital affiliated with the university). The organization's type may affect its structure. Exhibit 1-1 summarizes the subgroups of both proprietary and nonprofit organizations.

Organization Charts

In a small organization, top management will be able to see what is happening. Extensive measures and indicators are not necessary because management can view overall operations. But in a large organization, top management must use the management control system to understand what is going on. In other words, to view operations, management must use measures and indicators because he or she cannot get a firsthand overall picture of the total organization.

As a rule of thumb, an informal management control system is acceptable only if the manager can stay in close contact with all aspects of the operation. Otherwise, a formal

Exhibit 1–1 Types of Organizations

Profit Oriented—Proprietary
   Individual
   Partnership
   Corporation
   Other
Nonprofit—Voluntary
   Church Associated
   Private School Associated
   Foundation Associated
   Other
Nonprofit—Government
   Federal
   State
   County
   City
   City-County
   Hospital District
   State University
   Other

system is required. In the context of health care, therefore, a one-physician practice (Figure 1-2) could use an informal method, but a hospital system (Figure 1-3) must use a formal method of management control.

The structure of the organization will affect its financial management. Organization charts are often used to illustrate the structure of the organization. Each box on an organization chart represents a particular area of management responsibility. The lines between the boxes are lines of authority.

In the health system organization chart illustrated in Figure 1-3, the president/chief executive officer oversees seven senior vice-presidents. Each senior vice-president has vice-presidents reporting to him or her in each particular area of responsibility designated on the chart. These vice-presidents, in turn, have an array of other managers reporting to them at varying levels of managerial responsibility.

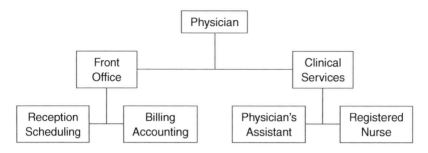

Figure 1–2 Physician's Office Organization Chart (Single Practitioner). Courtesy of Resource Group, Ltd., Dallas, Texas.

The organization chart also shows the degree of decentralization within the organization. Decentralization indicates the delegating of authority for decision making. The chart thus illustrates the pattern of how managers are allowed—or required—to make key decisions within the particular organization.

The purpose of an organization chart, then, is to indicate how responsibility is assigned to managers and to indicate the formal lines of communication and reporting.

TWO TYPES OF ACCOUNTING

Financial

Financial accounting is generally for outside, or third-party, use. Thus, financial accounting emphasizes external reporting. External reporting to third parties in health care includes, for example, government entities (Medicare, Medicaid, and other government programs) and health plan payers. In addition, proprietary organizations may have to report to stockholders, taxing district hospitals have to report to taxpayers, and so on.

Financial reporting for external purposes must be in accordance with generally accepted accounting principles. Financial reporting is usually concerned with transactions that have already occurred: that is, it is retrospective.

Managerial

Managerial accounting is generally for inside, or internal, use. Managerial accounting, as its title implies, is used by managers. The planning and control of operations and related performance measures are common day-by-day uses of managerial accounting. Likewise, the reporting of profitability of services and the pricing of services are other common ongoing uses of managerial accounting. Strategic planning and other intermediate and long-term decision making represent an additional use of managerial accounting.[3]

Managerial accounting intended for internal use is not bound by generally accepted accounting principles. Managerial accounting deals with transactions that have already occurred, but it is also concerned with the future, in the form of projecting outcomes and preparing budgets. Thus, managerial accounting is prospective as well as retrospective.

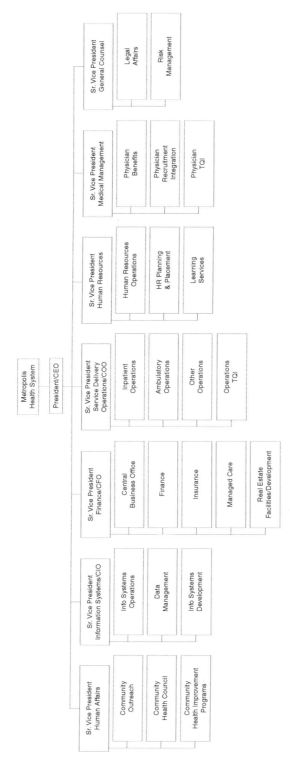

Figure 1–3 Health System Organization Chart. Courtesy of Resource Group, Ltd., Dallas, Texas.

INFORMATION CHECKPOINT

What Is Needed?	Reports for management purposes.
Where Is It Found?	With your supervisor.
How Is It Used?	To manage better.
What Is Needed?	Organization chart.
Where Is It Found?	With your supervisor or in the administrative offices.
How Is It Used?	To better understand the structure and lines of authority in your organization.

 KEY TERMS

Controlling
Decision Making
Financial Accounting
Managerial Accounting
Nonprofit Organization (also see *Voluntary Organization*)
Organization Chart
Organizing
Planning
Proprietary Organization (also see *Profit-Oriented Organization*)

 DISCUSSION QUESTIONS

1. What element of financial management do you perform most often in your job?
2. Do you perform all four elements? If not, why not?
3. Of the organization types described in this chapter, what type is the one you work for?
4. Have you ever seen your company's organization chart? If so, how decentralized is it?
5. If you receive reports in the course of your work, do you believe that they are prepared for outside (third-party) use or for internal (management) use? What leads you to believe this?

CHAPTER 2

What Does the Health Care Manager Need to Know?

PROGRESS NOTES

After completing this chapter, you should be able to

1. Understand that four segments make a financial management system work.
2. Follow an information flow.
3. Recognize the basic system elements.
4. Follow the annual management cycle.

HOW THE SYSTEM WORKS IN HEALTH CARE

The information that you, as a manager, work with is only one part of an overall system. To understand financial management, it is essential to recognize the overall system in which your organization operates. An order exists within the system, and it is generally up to you to find that order. Watch for how the information fits together. The four segments that make a health care financial system work are (1) the original records, (2) the information system, (3) the accounting system, (4) and the reporting system. Gen-erally speaking, the original records provide evidence that some event has occurred; the information system gathers this evidence; the accounting system records the evidence, and the reporting system produces reports of the effect. The health care manager needs to know that these separate elements exist and that they work together for an end result.

THE INFORMATION FLOW

Structure of the Information System

Information systems can be simplistic or highly complex. They can be fully auto-mated or semiautomated. Occasionally—even today—they can still be generated by hand and not by computer. (This last in-stance is becoming rare and can happen today only in certain small and relatively iso-lated health care organizations that are not yet required to electronically submit their billings.)

We will examine a particular information system and point out the basics that a man-ager should be able to recognize. Figure 2-1 shows information system components for an ambulatory care setting. This complex system uses a clinical and financial data repository; in other words, both clinical and

11

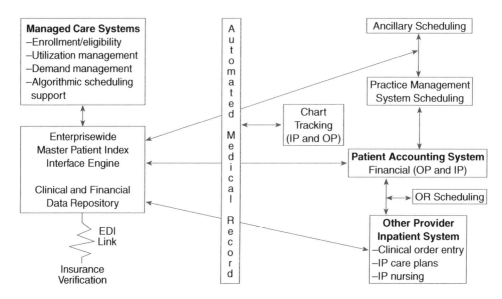

Figure 2–1 Information System Components for an Ambulatory Care Setting; OP, Outpatient; IP, Inpatient; OR, Operating Room.

financial data are fed into the same system. An automated medical record is also linked to the system. These are basic facts that a manager should recognize about this ambulatory information system.

In addition, the financial information, both outpatient and any relevant inpatient, is fed into the data repository. Scheduling-system data also enter the data repository, along with any relevant inpatient care plan and nursing information. Again, all of these are basic facts that a manager should recognize about this ambulatory care information system.

These items have all been inputs. One output from the clinical and financial data repository (also shown in Figure 2–1) is insurance verification for patients through an electronic data information (EDI) link to insurance company databases. Insurance verification is daily operating information. Another output is decision-making informa-

tion for managed care strategic planning, including support for demand, utilization, enrollment, and eligibility, plus some statistical support. The manager does not have to understand the specifics of all the inputs and outputs of this complex system, but he or she should recognize that these outputs occur when this ambulatory system is activated.

Function of Flowsheets

Flowsheets illustrate, as in this case, the flow of activities that capture information.[1] Flowsheets are useful because they portray who is responsible for what piece of information as it enters the system. The manager needs to realize the significance of such information. We give, as an example, obtaining confirmation of a patient's correct address. The manager should know that a correct address for a patient is vital to the smooth operation of the system. An incorrect address will, for example, cause the billing to be rejected. Understanding this connection between deficient data (e.g., a bad address) and the consequences (the bill will be rejected by the payer and thus not be paid) illustrates the essence of good financial management knowledge.

We can examine two examples of patient information flows. The first, shown in Figure 2-2, is a physician's office flowsheet for address confirmation. Four different personnel are involved in addition to the patient. This physician has computed the cost of a bad address as $12.30 to track down each address correction. He pays close attention to the handling of this information because he knows that there is a direct financial management consequence in his operation.

The second example, shown in Figure 2-3, is a health system flowsheet for verification of patient information. This flowsheet illustrates the process for a home care system. In this case, the flow begins not with a receptionist, as in the physician office example, but with a central database. This central database downloads the information and generates a summary report to be reviewed the next day. Appropriate verification is then made in a series of steps, and any necessary corrections are made before the form goes to the billing department. The object of the flow is the same in both examples: that is, the billing must have a correct address to receive payment. But the flow is different within two different systems. A manager must understand how the system works to understand the consequences. Then good financial management can prevail.

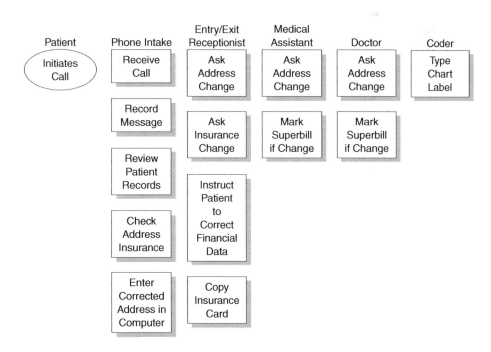

Figure 2–2 Physician's Office Flowsheet for Address Confirmation.

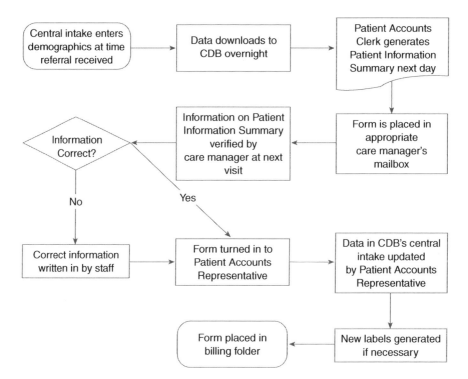

Figure 2–3 Health System Flowsheet for Verification of Patient Information.

BASIC SYSTEM ELEMENTS

To understand financial management, it is essential to decipher the reports provided to the manager. To comprehend these reports, it is helpful to understand certain basic system elements that are used to create the information contained in the reports.

Chart of Accounts—The Map

The chart of accounts is a map. It outlines the elements of your company in an organized manner. The chart of accounts maps out account titles with a method of numeric coding. It is designed to compile financial data in a uniform manner that the user can decode.

The groupings of accounts in the chart of accounts should match the groupings of the organization. In other words, the classification on the organization chart (as discussed in the previous chapter) should be compatible with the groupings on the chart of accounts. Thus, if there is a human resources department on your facility's organization chart and if expenses are grouped by department in your facility, then we would expect to find a human resources grouping in the chart of accounts.

The manager who is working with financial data needs to be able to read and comprehend how the dollars are laid out and how they are gathered together, or assembled. This assembly happens through the guidance of the chart of accounts. That is why we compare it to a map.

Basic guidance for health care charts of accounts is set out in publications such as that of Seawell's Chart of Accounts for Hospitals.[2] However, generic guides are just that—generic. Every organization exhibits differences in its own chart of accounts that express the unique aspects of its structure. We examine three examples to illustrate these differences. Remember, we are spending time on the chart of accounts because your comprehension of detailed financial data may well depend on whether you can decipher your facility's own chart of accounts mapping in the information forwarded for your use.

The first format, shown in Exhibit 2-1, is a basic use, probably for a smaller organization. The exhibit is in two horizontal segments, "Structure" and "Example." There

are three parts to the account number. The first part is one digit and indicates the financial statement element. Thus, our example shows "1," which is for "Asset." The second part is two digits and is the primary subclassification. Our example shows "10," which stands for "Current Asset" in this case. The third and final part is also two digits and is the secondary subclassification. Our example shows "11," which stands for "Petty Cash—Front Office" in this case. On a report, this account number would probably appear as 1-10-11.

The second format, shown in Exhibit 2-2, is full use and would be for a large organization. The exhibit is again in two horizontal segments, "Structure" and "Example," and there are now two line items appearing in the Example section. This full-use example has five parts to the account number. The first part is two digits and indicates the entity

---

Exhibit 2–1 Chart of Accounts, Format 1

Structure		
X	XX	XX
Financial Statement Element	Primary Subclassification	Secondary Subclassification

Example		
1	10	11
Asset	Current Asset	Petty Cash— Front Office
(Financial Statement Element)	(Primary Subclassification)	(Secondary Subclassification)

Exhibit 2–2 Chart of Accounts, Format 2

Structure				
XX	XX	X	XXXX	XX
Entity Designator	Fund Designator	Financial Statement Element	Primary Subclassification	Secondary Subclassification

Example				
10	10	4	3125	03
Hospital A	General Fund	Revenue	Lab—Microbiology	Payer: XYZ HMO
10	10	6	3125	10
Hospital A	General Fund	Expense	Lab—Microbiology	Clerical Salaries
(Entity Designator)	(Fund Designator)	(Financial Statement Element)	(Primary Subclassification)	(Secondary Subclassification)

designator number. Thus, we conclude that there is more than one entity within this system. Our example shows "10," which stands for "Hospital A." The second part is two digits and indicates the fund designator number. Thus, we conclude that there is more than one fund within this system. Our example shows "10," which stands for "General Fund."

The third part of Exhibit 2–2 is one digit and indicates the financial statement element. Thus, the first line of our example shows "4," which is for "Revenue," and the second line of our example shows "6," which is for "Expense." (The third part of this example is the first part of the simpler example shown in Exhibit 2-1.) The fourth part is four digits and is the primary subclassification. Our example shows "3125," which stands for "Lab—Microbiology." The num-

ber "3125" appears on both lines of this example, indicating that both the revenue and the expense belong to Lab—Microbiology. (The fourth part of this example is the second part of the simpler example shown in Exhibit 2-1. The simpler example used only two digits for this part, but this full-use example uses four digits.) The fifth and final part is two digits and is the secondary subclassification. Our example shows "03" on the first line, the revenue line, which stands for "Payer: XYZ HMO" and indicates the source of the revenue. On the second line, the expense line, our example shows "10," which stands for "Clerical Salaries." Therefore, we understand that these are the clerical salaries belonging to Lab—Microbiology in Hospital A. (The fifth part of this example is the third and final part of the simpler example shown in Exhibit 2-1.) On a report, these account numbers might appear as 10-10-4-3125-03 and 10-10-6-3125-10. Another optional use that is easier to read at a glance is 10104-3125-03 and 10106-3125-10.

Because every organization is unique and because the chart of accounts reflects that uniqueness, the third format, shown in Exhibit 2-3, illustrates a customized use of the chart of accounts. This example is adapted from a large hospital system. There are four parts to its chart of accounts number. The first part is an entity designator and designates a company within the hospital system. The fund designator two-digit part as traditionally used (see Exhibit 2-2) is missing here. The financial statement element one-digit part as traditionally used (see Exhibit 2-2) is also missing here. Instead, the second part of Exhibit 2-3 represents the primary classification, which is shown as an expense category ("Payroll") in the example line.

The third part of Exhibit 2-3 is the secondary subclassification, representing a labor subaccount expense designation ("Regular per-Visit RN"). The fourth and final part of Exhibit 2-3 is another subclassification that indicates the department within the company ("Home Health"). On a report for this organization, therefore, the account number 21-7000-2200-7151 would indicate the home care services company's payroll for regular per-visit registered nurses (RNs) in the home health department. Finally, remember that time spent understanding your own facility's chart of accounts will be time well spent.

Books and Records—Capture Transactions

The books and records of the financial information system for the organization serve

---

Exhibit 2–3 Chart of Accounts, Format 3

Structure			
XX	XXXX	XXXX	XXXX
Company	Expense Category	Subaccount	Department
(Entity Designator)	(Primary Classification)	(Secondary Subclassification)	(Additional Subclassification)

Example			
21	7000	2200	7151
Home Care Services	Payroll	Regular per-Visit RN	Home Health
(Company)	(Expense Category)	(Subaccount)	(Department)

to capture transactions. Figure 2-4 illustrates the relationship of the books and records to each other. As a single transaction occurs, the process begins. The individual transaction is recorded in the appropriate subsidiary journal. Similar such transactions are then grouped and balanced within the subsidiary journal. At periodic intervals, the groups of transactions are gathered, summarized, and entered in the general ledger. Within the general ledger, the transaction groups are reviewed and adjusted. After such review and adjustment, the transactions for the period within the general ledger are balanced. A document known as the trial balance is used for this purpose. The final step in the process is to create statements that reflect the transactions for the period. The trial balance is used to produce the statements.

All transactions for the period reside in the general ledger. The subsidiary journals are so named because they are "subsidiary" to the general ledger: in other words, they serve to support the general ledger. Figure 2-5 illustrates this concept. Another way to think of the subsidiary journals is to picture them as feeding the general ledger. The important point here is to understand the source and the flow of information as it is recorded.

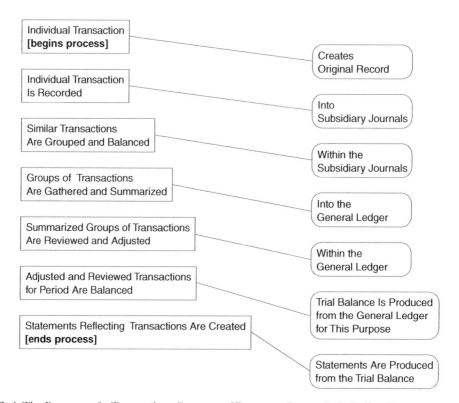

Figure 2–4 The Progress of a Transaction. Courtesy of Resource Group, Ltd., Dallas, Texas.

THE BOOKS

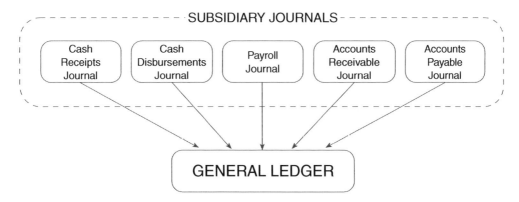

Figure 2–5 Recording Information: Relationship of Subsidiary Journals to the General Ledger. Courtesy of Resource Group, Ltd. Dallas, Texas.

Reports—The Product

Reports are more fully treated in a subsequent chapter of this text (see Chapter 9). It is sufficient at this point to recognize that reports are the final product of a process that commences with an original transaction.

THE ANNUAL MANAGEMENT CYCLE

The annual management cycle affects the type and status of information that the manager is expected to use. Some operating information is "raw"—that is, unadjusted. When the same information has passed further through the system and has been verified, adjusted, and balanced, it will usually vary from the initial raw data. These differences are a part of the process just described.

Daily and Weekly Operating Reports

The daily and weekly operating reports generally contain raw data, as discussed in the preceding paragraph. The purpose of such daily and weekly reports is to provide immediate operating information to use for day-by-day management purposes.

Quarterly Reports and Statistics

The quarterly reports and statistics generally have been verified, adjusted, and balanced. They are called *interim* reports because they have been generated sometime during the reporting period of the organization and not at the end of that period. Managers often used quarterly reports as milestones. A common milestone is the quarterly budget review.

Annual Year-End Reports

Most organizations have a 12-month reporting period known as a fiscal year. A fiscal year therefore covers a period from the first day of a particular month (e.g., January 1) through the last day of a month that is one year, or 12 months, in the future (e.g., December 31). If we see a heading that reads "For the year ended June 30," we know that the fiscal year began on July 1 of the previous year. Anything less than a full 12-month year is called a "stub period" and is fully spelled out in the heading. If, therefore, a company is reporting for a three-month stub period ending on December 31, the heading on the report will read, "For the threemonth period ended December 31." An alternative treatment uses a heading that reads, "For the period October 1 to December 31."

Annual year-end reports cover the full 12-month reporting period or the fiscal year. Such annual year-end reports are not primarily intended for managers' use. Their primary purpose is for reporting the operations of the organization for the period to outsiders, or third parties.

Annual year-end reports represent the closing out of the information system for a specific reporting period. The recording and reporting of operations will now begin a new cycle with a new year.

COMMUNICATING FINANCIAL INFORMATION TO OTHERS

The ability to communicate financial information effectively to others is a valuable skill. It is important to

- Create a report as your method of communication.
- Use accepted terminology.
- Use standard formats that are accepted in the accounting profession.
- Begin with an executive summary.
- Organize the body of the report in a logical flow.
- Place extensive detail into an appendix.

The rest of this book will help you learn how to create such a report. Our book will also sharpen your communication skills by helping you better understand how heath care finance works.

 INFORMATION CHECKPOINT

What Is Needed?	An explanation of how the information flow works in your unit.
Where Is It Found?	Probably with the information system staff; perhaps in the administrative offices.
How Is It Used?	Study the flow and relate it to the paperwork that you handle.

 KEY TERMS

Accounting System
Chart of Accounts
General Ledger
Information System
Original Records
Reporting System
Subsidiary Journals
Trial Balance

DISCUSSION QUESTIONS

1. Have you ever been informed of the information flow in your unit or division?
2. If so, did you receive the information in a formal seminar or in an informal manner, one on one with another individual? Do you think this was the best way? Why?
3. Do you know about the chart of accounts in your organization as it pertains to information you receive?
4. If so, is it similar to one of the three formats illustrated in this chapter? If not, how is it different?
5. Do you work with daily or weekly operating reports? With quarterly reports and statistics?
6. If so, do these reports give you useful information? How do you think they could be improved?

PART II

Record Financial Operations

CHAPTER 3

Assets, Liabilities, and Net Worth

PROGRESS NOTES

After completing this chapter you should be able to

1. Recognize typical assets.
2. Recognize typical liabilities.
3. Understand net worth terminology.
4. See how assets, liabilities, and net worth fit together.

OVERVIEW

Assets, liabilities, and net worth are part of the language of finance. As such, it is important to understand both their composition and how they fit together. Short definitions appear below, followed by examples.

Assets

Assets are economic resources that have expected future benefits to the business. In other words, assets are what the organization owns and/or controls.

Liabilities

Liabilities are "outsider claims" consisting of economic obligations, or debts, payable to outsiders. Thus, liabilities are what the organization owes, and the outsiders to whom the debts are due are creditors of the business.

Net Worth

"Insider claims" are called owner's equity, or net worth. These are claims held by the owners of the business. An owner has a claim to the entity's assets because he or she has invested in the business. No matter what term is used, the sum of these claims reflects what the business is worth, net of liabilities—thus "net worth."

The Three-Part Equation

An accounting equation reflects a relationship among assets, liabilities, and net worth as follows: assets equal liabilities plus net worth. The three pieces must always balance among themselves because this is how they fit together. The equation is as follows:

$$\text{Assets} = \text{Liabilities} + \text{Net Worth.}$$

WHAT ARE EXAMPLES OF ASSETS?

All of the following are typical business assets.

Examples of Assets

Cash, accounts receivable, notes receivable, and inventory are all assets. If the Great Lakes Home Health Agency (HHA) has cash in its bank account, that is an economic resource—an asset. The HHA is owed money for services rendered; these accounts receivable are also an economic resource—an asset. If certain patients have signed a formal agreement to pay the HHA, then these notes receivable are likewise economic resources—assets. All types of business receivables are assets. The Great Lakes HHA also has an inventory of medical supplies (dressings, syringes, IV tubing, etc.) that are used in its day-to-day operations. This inventory on hand is an economic resource—an asset. Land, buildings, and equipment are also assets. Exhibit 3-1 summarizes asset examples.

Short-Term Versus Long-Term Assets

Assets are often labeled either "current" or "long-term" assets. "Current" is another word for "short-term." If an asset can be turned into cash within a 12-month period, it is current, or short term. If, on the other hand, an asset cannot be converted into cash within a 12-month period, it is considered

---

Exhibit 3–1 Asset Examples

Cash
Accounts receivable
Notes receivable
Inventory
Land
Buildings
Equipment

---

long term. In our Great Lakes HHA example, accounts receivable should be collected within one year and thus should be current assets. Likewise, the inventory should be converted to business use within one year; thus, it too is considered short term.

Classification of the note receivable depends on the length of time that payment is promised. If the entire note receivable will be paid within one year, it is a short-term asset. Consider, however, what would happen if the note is to be paid over three years. A portion of the note—that amount to be paid in the coming 12 months—will be classified as short term or current, and the rest of the note—that amount to be paid further in the future—will be classified as long term.

The land, building, and equipment will generally be classified as long term because these assets will not be converted into cash in the coming 12 months. Buildings and equipment are also generally stated at a net figure called book value, which reduces their historical cost by any accumulated depreciation. (The concept of depreciation is discussed in Chapter 5.)

WHAT ARE EXAMPLES OF LIABILITIES?

All of the following are typical business liabilities.

Examples of Liabilities

Accounts payable, payroll taxes due, notes payable, and mortgages payable are all liabilities. The Great Lakes HHA owes vendors for medical supplies it has purchased. The amount owed to the vendors is recognized as accounts payable. When the HHA paid its employees, it withheld payroll taxes, as required by the government. The payroll taxes withheld are due to be paid to the government and thus are also a liability. The

HHA has borrowed money and signed a formal agreement, and thus, the amount due is a liability. The HHA also has a mortgage on its building. This mortgage is likewise a liability. In other words, debts are liabilities. Exhibit 3-2 summarizes liability examples.

Short-Term Versus Long-Term Liabilities

Liabilities are also usually labeled as either "current" (short term) or "long-term" liabilities. In this case, if a liability is expected to be paid within a 12-month period, it is current, or short term. If, however, the liability cannot reasonably be expected to be paid within a 12-month period, it is considered long term. In our Great Lakes HHA example, accounts payable and payroll taxes due should be paid within one year and thus should be labeled as current liabilities.

Classification of the note payable depends on the length of time that payment is promised. If the HHA is going to pay the entire note payable within one year, it is a short-term liability. But consider what would happen if the note is to be paid over three years. A portion of the note—that amount to be paid in the coming 12 months—will be classified as short term or current, and the rest of the note—that amount to be paid further in the future—will be classified as long term. The mortgage will be treated slightly differently. That portion to be paid within the coming 12 months will be classified as a short-term liability while the remaining mortgage balance will be labeled as long term.

WHAT ARE THE DIFFERENT FORMS OF NET WORTH?

Net worth—the third part of the accounting equation—is labeled differently depending on the type of organization. For-profit organizations will have equity accounts with which to report their net worth. (Equity is the ownership right in property or the money value of property.) For example, a sole proprietorship or a partnership's net worth may simply be labeled as "Owners' Equity." A corporation, on the other hand, will generally report two types of equity accounts: "Capital Stock" and "Retained Earnings." Capital Stock represents the owners' investment in the company, indicated by their purchase of stock. Retained Earnings, as the name implies, represents undistributed company income that has been left in the business.

Not-for-profit organizations will generally use a different term such as "Fund Balance" to report the difference between assets and liabilities in their report. This is presumably because nonprofits should not, by definition, have equity. Exhibit 3-3 summarizes terminology examples for net worth as just discussed.

Exhibit 3–2 Liability Examples

Accounts payable
Payroll taxes due
Notes payable
Mortgage payable
Bonds payable

Exhibit 3–3 Net Worth Terminology Examples

For-profit sole proprietors or partnerships:
    Owners' Equity
For-profit corporations:
    Capital Stock
    Retained Earnings
Not-for-profit (nonprofit) companies:
    Fund Balance

INFORMATION CHECKPOINT

What Is Needed?	A report that shows the balance sheet for your organization.
Where Is It Found?	Probably with your supervisor.
How Is It Used?	Study the balance sheet to find the assets and liabilities. Check the equity section to see whether equity is listed as net worth or as fund balance.

 KEY TERMS

Assets
Equity
Fund Balance
Liabilities
Net Worth

 DISCUSSION QUESTIONS

1. Do you ever work with balance sheets in your current position?
2. If so, is the balance sheet you receive for your department only or for the entire organization? Do you know why this reporting method (departmental versus entire organization) was chosen by management?
3. If you receive a copy of the balance sheet, is one distributed to you once a month, once a year, or on some other more irregular basis? What are you supposed to do with it upon receipt?
4. Do you think the balance sheet report you receive gives you useful information? How do you think it could be improved?

Revenues (Inflow)

OVERVIEW

Revenue represents amounts earned by an organization: that is, actual or expected cash inflows due to the organization's major business. In the case of health care, revenue is mostly earned by rendering services to patients. Revenue flows into the organization and is sometimes referred to as the *revenue stream*.

Revenue is generally defined as the value of services rendered, expressed at the facility's full established rates. For example, hos-pital A's full established rate for a certain procedure is $100, but Giant Health Plan has negotiated a managed care contract whereby the plan pays only $90 for that procedure. The revenue figure—the full established rate—is $100. Revenues can be received in the form of cash or credit. Most, but not all, health care revenues are received in the form of credit.

RECEIVING REVENUE FOR SERVICES

One way that revenue is classified is by whether payment is received before or after the service is delivered. The amount of revenue received for services is often influenced by this classification.

Payment after Service Is Delivered

The traditional payment method in health care is that of payment after service is delivered. Two basic types of payment after service is delivered are discussed in this section: fee for service and discounted fee for service. One evolved from the other.

1. *Fee for service.* The truly traditional U.S. method of receiving revenue for serv-

ices is fee for service. The provider of services is paid according to the service performed. Before the 1970s, with a very few exceptions, fee for service was the dominant method of payment for health services in the United States.[1]

2. *Discounted fee for service.* In this variation on the original fee for service, a contracted discount is agreed upon. The organization providing the services then receives a payment that is discounted in accordance with the contract. Sometimes the contract contains fee schedules. A large provider of services can have many different contracts, all with different discounted contractual arrangements. Many variations are therefore possible.

Payment Before Service Is Delivered

Traditional payment methods in the United States have begun to give way to payment before service is delivered. There are multiple names and definitions for such payment. We have chosen to use a general descriptive term for payment received before service is delivered: *predetermined per-person payment.* The payment method itself and its rate-setting variations are discussed in this section.

1. *Predetermined per-person payment.* Payment received before service is delivered is generally at an agreed-upon predetermined rate. Payment therefore consists of the predetermined rate for each person covered under the agreement. Thus, the amount received is per-head or per-person count at a particular point in time.

2. *Rate-setting differences.* Different agreements can use varying assumptions about the group to be served, and these variations will affect the rate-setting process. Numerous variations are therefore possible.

Contractual Allowances and Other Deductions from Revenue

Revenues are recorded at the organization's full established rates, as previously discussed. Those amounts estimated to be uncollectible are considered to be deductions from revenues and are recorded as such on the books of the organization. (For purposes of the external financial statements released for third-party use, reported revenue must represent the amounts that payers [or patients] are obligated to pay. Therefore, the terms *gross revenue* and *deductions from revenue* will not be seen on external statements. The discussion that follows, however, pertains to the books and records that are used for internal management, where these classifications will be used.)

Contractual allowances are the difference between the full established rate and the agreed-upon contractual rate that will be paid. Contractual allowances are often for composite services. Take the case of hospital A as an example. As discussed in the overview to this chapter, hospital A's full established rate for a certain procedure is $100, but Giant Health Plan has negotiated a managed care contract whereby the plan pays only $90 for that procedure. The $10 difference between the revenue figure ($100) and the contracted amount that the plan pays ($90) represents the contractual allowance.

It is not uncommon for different plans to pay different contractual rates for the same service. This practice is illustrated in Table 4–1, which shows contractual rates to be paid

Table 4–1 Variations in Physician Office Revenue for Two Visit Codes

	Visit Codes	
Payer	99213	99214
FHP	$25.35	$35.70
HPHP	42.45	58.85
MC	39.05	54.90
UND	39.90	60.40
CCN	44.00	70.20
MAYO	45.75	70.75
CGN	10.00	10.00
PRU	39.05	54.90
PHCS	45.00	50.00
ANA	38.25	45.00

Rates for illustration only.

for visit codes 99213 and 99214 for 10 different health plans. Note the variations in rates.

The second major deduction from revenue classification is an allowance for bad debts, also known as a provision for doubtful accounts. (Again, for purposes of the external financial statements released for third-party use, the provision for doubtful reports must be reported separately as an expense item. The discussion that follows, however, still pertains to the books and records that are used for internal management, where the classification of deductions from revenue will be used.) The allowance for bad debts is charged with the amount of services received on credit (recorded as accounts receivable) that are estimated to result in credit losses.

Beyond contractual allowances and a provision for bad debts, the third major deduction from revenue classification is charity service. Charity service is generally defined as services provided to financially indigent patients.

SOURCES OF HEALTH CARE REVENUE

Health care revenue in the United States comes from a variety of public programs (governmental sources) and private payers. The sources of health care revenue are generally termed *payers*. Payer mix—the proportion of revenues realized from the different types of payers—is a measure that is often included in the profile of a health care organization. For example, "Hospital A has a payer mix that includes 40 percent Medicare and 33 percent Medicaid" might be part of the profile.

Governmental Sources

The Medicare Program

Title XVIII of the Social Security Act is commonly known as Medicare. Actually entitled "Health Insurance for the Aged and Disabled," Medicare legislation established a health insurance program for the aged in 1965. The program was intended to complement other benefits (such as retirement, survivors', and disability insurance benefits) under other titles within the Social Security Act.

The Medicare program has two parts. One, known as Part A, is hospital insurance (HI) and is funded primarily by a mandatory payroll tax. The other part, known as Part B, is called supplementary medical insurance (SMI). SMI is voluntary and is funded primarily by insurance premiums (usually deducted from monthly Social Security benefit checks of those enrolled), supplemented by federal general revenue funds. Guidelines determine both the services to be covered and the eligibility of the individual to receive the services under the Medicare program. Medicare claims (billings) are processed by fiscal agents who act on behalf of the federal government. These fiscal agents are known as *intermediaries* and *carriers*. Intermediaries process the claims for Part A (HI) institutional services and outpatient claims for Part B (SMI). Carriers process the claims for Part B (SMI) physician and medical supplier services.

Medicare's third part, Part C, is known as "Medicare Advantage." Medicare Advantage consists of managed care plans, private fee-for-service plans, preferred provider organization plans, and specialty plans. Although Medicare Advantage is offered as an alternative to traditional Medicare, coverage must never be less than what Part A and Part B (tradition Medicare) would offer the beneficiary. Medicare's fourth part, Part D, is the Prescription Drug Benefit, effective as of January 1, 2006. The prescription drug benefit represents expanded coverage. It is a voluntary program that requires payment of a separate premium and contains cost-sharing provisions.

The Medicare program covers approximately 95 percent of the U.S. aged population along with certain eligible individuals receiving Social Security disability benefits.[2] Medicare is an important source of health care revenue to most health care organizations.

The Medicaid Program

Title XIX of the Social Security Act is commonly known as Medicaid. Medicaid legislation established a federal and state matching entitlement program in 1965. The program was intended to provide medical assistance to eligible needy individuals and families.

The Medicaid program is state specific. The federal government has established broad national guidelines. Each state has the power to set eligibility, service restrictions, and payment rates for services within that state. In doing so, each state is bound only by the broad national guidelines. Medicaid policies are complex, and considerable variation exists among states. The federal government is responsible for a certain percentage of each state's Medicaid expenditures; the specific amount due is calculated by an annual formula. The state pays the providers of Medicaid services directly. Thus, the source of Medicaid revenue to a health care organization is considered to be the state government's Medicaid program representatives.

The Medicaid program is the largest U.S. government program providing funds for medical and health-related services for the poor.[3] Therefore, although the proportion of Medicaid services within the payer mix may vary, Medicaid is a source of health care revenue in almost every health care organization.

Other Programs

There are numerous other sources of federal, state, and local revenues for health care organizations. Generally speaking, for most organizations, none of the other revenue sources will exceed the Title XVIII and Title XIX programs just discussed. Other programs include the Department of Veterans' Affairs health programs, workers' compensation programs, and state-only general assistance programs (versus the federal-and-state jointly funded Medicaid program). Still other public programs are school health programs, public health clinics, maternal and child health services, migrant health care services, certain mental health and drug and alcohol services, and special programs such as Indian health care services.

Managed Care Sources

In the 1970s, managed care began to appear in health care models in the United States. An all-purpose definition of managed care is: managed care is a means of providing health care services within a network of health care providers. The responsibility to manage and provide high-quality and cost-effective health care is delegated to this defined network of providers.[4] A central concept of managed care is the coordination of all health care services for an individual. In general, managed care plans receive a predetermined amount per member in premiums.

Types of Plans

The most prevalent type of managed care plan today is the health maintenance organization (HMO). Members enroll in the HMO. They prepay a fixed monthly amount; in return, they receive comprehensive health services. The members must use the providers who are designated by the HMO; if they go outside the designated providers, they must pay all or a large part of the cost themselves. The designated providers of services in turn contract with the HMO to provide services at agreed-upon rates. Several different forms of HMOs have evolved over time.

The preferred provider organization (PPO) is a type of plan found across the United States. It consists of a group of providers called a panel. The panel members are an approved group of various types of providers, including hospitals and physicians. The panel is limited in size and generally has utilization review powers. If the patients in a PPO use health providers who are not within the PPO itself, they must pay a higher amount in deductibles and coinsurance.

Types of Contracts

In the case of an HMO, the designated providers of health services contract with the HMO to provide services at agreed-upon rates. The different types of HMOs—including the staff model, the group model, the network model, the point-of-service model, and the individual practice association (IPA) model—have various methods of arriving at these rates. A PPO contracts with its selected group, who are all participating payers, to buy services for its eligible beneficiaries on the basis of discounted fee for service. A large health care facility will have one or more individuals responsible for managed care contracting.[5]

Other Revenue Sources

A considerable amount of health care revenues is still realized from sources other than Title XVIII, Title XIX, and managed care:

- *Commercial insurers.* Generally speaking, conventional indemnity insurers, or commercial insurers, simply pay for the eligible health services used by those individuals who pay premiums for health care insurance. They do not tend to have a say in how those health services are administered.
- *Private pay.* This is payment by patients themselves or by the families of patients. Private pay is more prevalent in nursing facilities and in assisted-living facilities than in hospital settings. Physicians' offices also receive a certain amount of private pay revenue.
- *Other.* Additional sources of revenue for health care facilities include donations received by voluntary nonprofit organizations and tax revenues levied

by governmental nonprofit organizations.

Health care revenue is often reported to managers by source of the revenue. Table 4–2 presents such a revenue summary. This example covers all types of sources discussed in this section. Both dollar totals and proportionate percentages by source are reported.

GROUPING REVENUE FOR PLANNING AND CONTROL

Grouping revenue by different classifications is an effective method for managers to use the information to plan and to control. In the preceding paragraph, we have just seen revenue reported by source. Other classification examples are now discussed.

Revenue Centers

A revenue center classification is one form of a responsibility center. In a responsibility center, the manager is responsible, as the name implies, for a particular set of activities. In the case of a revenue center, a par-

ticular unit of the organization is given responsibility for generating revenues to meet a certain target. Actually, the responsibility in the health care setting is more for generating volume than for generating a specific revenue dollar amount. (The implication is that the volume will, in turn, generate the dollars.) Revenue centers tend to occur most often in special programs where volume is critical to survival of the program.

Care Settings

Grouping revenue by care setting recognizes the different sites at which services are delivered. The most basic grouping by care settings is inpatient versus ambulatory services. Exhibit 4–1, however, illustrates a six-way classification of care setting revenues within a health system. In this case, hospital inpatient, hospital outpatient, off-site clinic, skilled nursing facility, home health agency, and hospice are all accounted for. A percentage is shown for each. This type of classification is useful for a brochure or a report that profiles the different types of health care services offered by the organization.

Table 4–2 Sample Monthly Statement of Revenue by Source

Summary	Year to Date	%
Private revenue	$100,000	2.9
HMO revenue	560,000	16.7
Medicare revenue	1,420,000	42.4
Medicaid revenue	820,000	24.5
Commercial revenue	400,000	12.0
Other revenue	50,000	1.5
Total	$3,350,000	100.0%

Exhibit 4–1 Revenues by Care Setting

42% Hospital Inpatient	38% Hospital Outpatient	4% Off-Site Clinic
8% Skilled Nursing Facility	6% Home Health Agency	2% Hospice

Service Lines

In traditional cost accounting circles, a product line is a grouping of similar products.[6] In the health care field, many organizations opt instead for "service line" terminology. A service line is a grouping of similar services. Strategic planning sometimes sets out service lines.

Hospitals

A number of hospitals have adopted the major diagnostic categories (MDCs) as service lines. One advantage of MDCs is that they are a universal designation in the United States. MDCs also have the advantage of possessing a standard definition. In another approach to service line classification, a hospital recently updated its strategic plan and settled on five service lines: (1) medical, (2) surgical, (3) women and children, (4) mental health, and (5) rehabilitation (neuro ortho rehab) (see Figure 4–1).

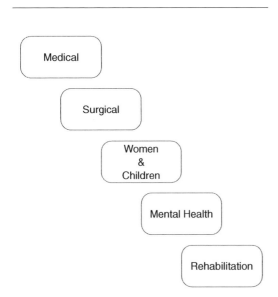

Figure 4–1 Hospital Service Lines. Courtesy of Resource Group, Ltd., Dallas, Texas.

Long-Term Care

A continuing care retirement community (CCRC) can use its various levels of care as a starting point. Thus, the CCRC usually has four service lines, listed in the descending order of resident acuity: (1) skilled nursing facility, (2) nursing facility, (3) assisted living, and (4) independent living. The skilled nursing facility provides services for the highest level of resident acuity, and the independent living provides services for the lowest level of resident acuity. One adjustment to this approach includes isolating subacute services from the remainder of skilled nursing facility services. Another adjustment involves splitting independent living into two categories, one for Housing and Urban Development (HUD)–subsidized independent housing and the other for private-pay independent housing. Figure 4–2 illustrates CCRC service lines by acuity level.

Home Care

Numerous categories of service delivery can be considered as "home care." A practical approach was taken by one home care entity—part of a health system—that defined its "key functions." Key functions can in turn be converted to service lines (Figure 4–3).

Physician Groups

Service delivery for physician groups will vary, of course, with the nature of the group itself. A generic set of service lines is presented in Figure 4–4.

Other Designations

Other classifications may meet the needs of particular organizations. Columbia/HCA is now reported to classify its services in a disease management approach. The classifica-

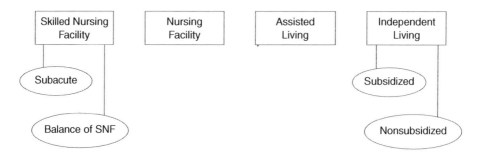

Figure 4–2 Long-Term Care Service Lines. Courtesy of Resource Group, Ltd., Dallas, Texas.

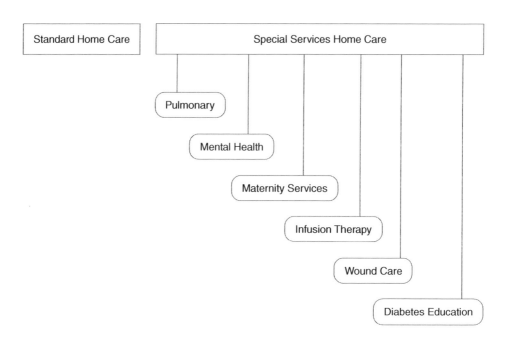

Figure 4–3 Home Care Service Lines. Courtesy of Resource Group, Ltd., Dallas, Texas.

tion consists of eight disease management areas: (1) cancer, (2) cardiology, (3) diabetes, (4) behavioral health, (5) workers' compensation, (6) women's services, (7) senior care, and (8) emergency services.[7] Whatever classification is chosen, it must be consistent with the current structure of the organization.

Office Visits

Surgical
Procedures

Emergency
Medicine

Laboratory

Radiology

Figure 4–4 Physicians Group Service Lines. Courtesy of Resource Group, Ltd., Dallas, Texas.

 INFORMATION CHECKPOINT

What Is Needed?	A report that shows revenue in your organization.
Where Is It Found?	With your supervisor.
How Is It Used?	Examine the report to find various revenue sources; look for how the contractual allowances and discounts are handled on the report.
What Is Needed?	A report that groups revenue by some type of classification.
Where Is It Found?	With your supervisor, or in the information services division.
How Is It Used?	Examine the report to discover the methods that are used for grouping. You will probably find that these groupings are used for performance measures. They can also be used for control and planning.

 KEY TERMS

Discounted Fee for Service
Fee for Service
Managed Care
Medicaid Program
Medicare Program
Payer Mix
Revenue

DISCUSSION QUESTIONS

1. Does your organization receive revenue mainly in the form of payment after service is delivered or payment before service is delivered?
2. Why do you think this is so?
3. What do you believe the proportion of revenues from different sources is for your organization?
4. Do you believe that this proportion (payer mix) will change in the future? Why?
5. What grouping of revenue do you believe your organization uses (revenue centers, care settings, service lines, other)?
6. From your perspective, would there be a better grouping possible? If so, why do you think it is not used?

CHAPTER 5

Expenses (Outflow)

PROGRESS NOTES

After completing this chapter, you should be able to

1. Understand the distinction between expense and cost.
2. Understand how disbursements for services represent an expense stream (an outflow).
3. Follow how expenses are grouped in different ways for planning and control.
4. Recognize why cost reports have influenced expense formats.

OVERVIEW

Expenses are the costs that relate to the earning of revenue. Another way to think of expenses is as the costs of doing business. Just as revenues represent the inflow into the organization, so do expenses represent the outflow—a stream of expenditures flowing out of the organization. Examples of expenses include salary expense for labor performed, payroll tax expense for taxes paid on the salary, utility expense for electricity, and interest expense for the use of money.

In actual fact, expenses are expired costs—costs that have been used up, or consumed, while carrying on business. Revenues and expenses affect the equity of the business. The inflow of revenues increases equity, whereas the outflow of expenses decreases equity. In nonprofit organizations, the term is *fund balance* rather than *equity*. This is because a nonprofit organization, by its nature, is not in business to make a profit. Thus, it should not have equity. However, the principle of inflow and outflow remains the same. In the case of nonprofits, the inflow of revenues increases fund balance, and the outflow of expenses decreases fund balance.

Many managers use the terms *expense* and *cost* interchangeably. *Expense* in its broadest sense includes every expired (used-up) cost that is deductible from revenue. A narrower interpretation groups expenses into categories such as operating expenses, administrative expenses, and so on. *Cost* is the amount of cash expended (or property transferred, services performed, or liability incurred) in consideration of goods or services received or to be received. As we have already said, costs can be either expired or unexpired. Expired costs are used up in the current period and are thus matched against current revenues. Unexpired costs are not yet used up and will be matched against future revenues.[1]

For example, an electric bill for $500 is recorded in the books of the clinic as an expense. The administrator sees the $500 as the cost of electricity for that month in the clinic. And the administrator is actually correct in seeing the $500 as a cost because it has been used up (expired) within the month.

Confusion also exists in health care reporting over the term *cost* versus *charges*. Charges are revenue, or inflow. Costs are expenses, or outflow. Charges add; costs take away. Because the two are inherently different, they should never be intermingled.

DISBURSEMENTS FOR SERVICES

There are two types of disbursements for services:

1. *Payment when expense is incurred.* If an expense is paid for at the point where it is incurred, it does not enter the accounts payable account. In large organizations, it is relatively rare to see payments when expenses are incurred. The only place where this usually occurs is the petty cash fund.

2. *Payment after expense is incurred.* In most health care organizations, expenses are paid at a later time and not at the point when the expense is incurred. If this is the case, the expense is recorded in accounts payable account. It is cleared from accounts payable when payment is made. One measurement of operations is "days in accounts payable," whereby the operating expenses for the organization are reduced to a rate per day and compared with the amount in accounts payable.

GROUPING EXPENSES FOR PLANNING AND CONTROL

Cost Centers

A cost center is one form of a responsibility center. In a responsibility center, the manager is responsible, as the name implies, for a particular set of activities. In the case of a cost center, a particular unit of the organization is given responsibility for controlling costs of the operations over which it holds authority. The medical records division is an example of a cost center. The billing and collection office might be another example. A cost center might be a division, an office, or an entire department, depending on how the organization is structured.

In health care organizations, it is common to find departments as cost centers. This is often a logical way to designate a cost center because the lines of authority are generally organized by department. Cost centers can then be grouped into larger groups that have something in common. Within this method of grouping, the manager of a cost center may receive his or her own reports and figures but not those of the entire group. The director or officer that is in charge of all of those particular departments receives the larger report that contains multiple cost centers. The chief executive officer receives a total report because he or she is ultimately responsible for overseeing the operations of all of the cost centers involved in that segment of the organization.

Exhibit 5–1 illustrates this concept. It contains 20 different cost centers, all of which are revenue producing. The 20 cost centers are divided into two groups: nursing services and other professional services. There are five cost centers in the nursing services group, ranging from operating

Exhibit 5–1 Nursing Services and Other Professional Services Cost Centers

Nursing Services Cost Center	
Nursing Services	
Routine Medical-Surgical	$390,000
Operating Room	30,000
Intensive Care Units	40,000
OB-Nursery	15,000
Other	35,000
Total	$510,000

Other Professional Services Cost Center	
Other Professional Services	
Laboratory	$220,000
Radiology	139,000
CT Scanner	18,000
Pharmacy	128,000
Emergency Service	89,000
Medical and Surgical Supply	168,000
Operating Rooms and Anesthesia	142,000
Respiratory Therapy	48,000
Physical Therapy	64,000
EKG	16,000
EEG	1,000
Ambulance Service	7,000
Substance Abuse	43,000
Home Health and Hospice	120,000
Other	12,000
Total	$1,215,000

Exhibit 5–2 General service and Support Services Cost Centers

General Services Cost Center	
General Services	
Dietary	$97,000
Maintenance	92,000
Laundry	27,000
Housekeeping	43,000
Security	5,000
Medical Records	30,000
Total	$294,000

Support Services Cost Center	
Support Services	
General	$455,000
Insurance	24,000
Social Security Taxes	112,000
Employee Welfare	188,000
Pension	43,000
Total	$822,000

room to obstetrics–nursery. There are 15 cost centers in the other professional services group. In the hospital that uses the grouping shown in Exhibit 5–1, however, not all of the 20 cost centers are departments. Some are divisions within departments. For example, EKG and EEG operate out of the same department but are two separate cost centers.

Exhibit 5–2 shows 11 different cost centers that are *not* directly revenue producing.

(The dietary department yields some cafeteria revenue, but that revenue is not central to the major business of the organization, which is to provide health care services.) The 11 cost centers are divided into two groups: general services and support services. The six cost centers in the general services group happen to all be departments in this hospital. (Other hospitals might not have security as a separate department. The other cost centers—dietary, maintenance, laundry, housekeeping, and medical records—would be separate departments.) The five cost centers in the support services group include one "general" cost center that contains administrative costs; the remaining four are related to employee salaries and wages. These four are insurance, social security taxes, employee welfare, and pension cost centers, all of which will probably be in the same department. It is the prerogative of management to set up cost centers specific to the organization's own needs and preferences. It is the responsibility of management to make the cost centers match the proper lines of authority.

Exhibit 5–2 illustrates two categories of health care expense: general services and support. A third related category is operations expense. An operations expense provides service directly related to patient care. Examples are radiology expense and drug expense. A general services expense provides services necessary to maintain the patient, but the service is not directly related to patient care. Examples are laundry and dietary. Support services expenses, on the other hand, provide support to both general services expenses and operations expenses. A support service expense is necessary for support, but it is neither directly related to patient care nor is it a service necessary to maintain the patient. Examples of support services are insurance and payroll taxes.

Diagnoses and Procedures

It is common to group expenses by diagnoses and procedures for purposes of planning and control. This grouping is beneficial because it matches costs against common classifications of revenues. Much of the revenue in many health care organizations is designated by either diagnoses or procedures. One prevalent method groups costs into cost centers by major diagnostic categories (MDCs). The 23 MDCs serve as the basic classification system for diagnosis-related groups (DRGs). (Each DRG represents a category of patients. This category contains patients whose resource consumption, on statistical average, is equivalent. DRGs are part of the prospective payment reimbursement methodology.) Exhibit 5–3 provides a listing of the 23 MDCs.

Exhibit 5–3 Major Diagnostic Categories

MDC 1	Diseases and Disorders of the Nervous System
MDC 2	Eye
MDC 3	Ear, Nose, Mouth, and Throat
MDC 4	Respiratory System
MDC 5	Circulatory System
MDC 6	Digestive System
MDC 7	Hepatobiliary System and Pancreas
MDC 8	Musculoskeletal System and Connective Tissue
MDC 9	Skin, Subcutaneous Tissue, and Breast
MDC 10	Endocrine, Nutritional, and Metabolic
MDC 11	Kidney and Urinary Tract
MDC 12	Male Reproductive System
MDC 13	Female Reproductive System
MDC 14	Pregnancy, Childbirth, and the Puerperium
MDC 15	Newborns and Other Neonates with Conditions Originating in the Perinatal Period
MDC 16	Blood and Blood-Forming Organs and Immunological Disorders
MDC 17	Myeloproliferative and Poorly and Differentiated Neoplasms
MDC 18	Infections and Parasitic Diseases (Systemic or Unspecified Sites)
MDC 19	Mental Diseases and Disorders
MDC 20	Alcohol/Drug Use and Alcohol/Drug-Induced Organic Mental Disorders
MDC 21	Injuries, Poisoning, and Toxic Effect of Drugs
MDC 22	Burns
MDC 23	Factors Influencing Health Status and Other Contacts with Health Services

How does the hospital use the MDC grouping? Exhibit 5–4 shows a departmental and cost center grouping in actual use. This hospital uses 27 cost center codes: the 23 MDCs plus four other codes ("Special Drugs," "HIV," "Unassigned," and "Outpatient"). The special drugs and HIV cost centers represent high-cost elements that management wants to track separately. "Unassigned" is a defaul category and should

have little assigned to it. "Outpatient" is a separate cost center at the preference of management.

Exhibit 5–5 illustrates the grouping of costs for MDC 18 (Infectious Diseases). Eighteen is the hospital's departmental code, per Exhibit 5–4. The DRG classification, ranging from 415 to 423, appears in the next column. The description of the particular DRG appears in the third column, and the related cost appears in the fourth and final column. These costs can now be readily matched to equivalent revenues.

Outpatient services in particular are generally designated by procedure codes. Procedure codes, known as Physicians' Current Procedural Terminology (CPT) codes, are commonly used to group cost centers for outpatient services. (CPT codes represent a listing of descriptive terms and identifying codes for identifying medical services and procedures performed.) However, procedures can—and are—also used for purposes of grouping inpatient costs, generally within a certain cost center. A hospital example of reporting radiology department costs by procedure code appears in Table 5–1. In this example, the procedure code is in the left column, the description of the procedure is in the middle column, and the departmental cost for the particular procedure appears in the right column. These costs can now be readily matched to equivalent revenue.

Care Settings and Service Lines

Expenses can be grouped by care setting, which recognizes the different sites at which services are delivered. "Inpatient" versus "outpatient" is a basic type of care setting grouping. Or expenses can be classified by service lines, a method that groups similar services.[2]

Exhibit 5–4 Hospital Departmental Code List Based on Major Diagnostic Categories

1	Nervous System
2	Eye
3	Ear, Nose, Mouth, and Throat
4	Respiratory System
5	Circulatory System
6	Digestive System
7	Hepatobiliary System
8	Musculoskeletal System and Connective Tissue
9	Skin, Subcutaneous Tissue, and Breast
10	Endocrine, Nutritional, and Metabolic
11	Kidney and Urinary Tract
12	Male Reproductive System
13	Female Reproductive System
14	Obstetrics
15	Newborns
16	Immunology
17	Oncology
18	Infectious Diseases
19	Mental Diseases
20	Substance Use
21	Injury, Poison, and Toxin
22	Burns
23	Other Health Services
24	Special Drugs
25	HIV
26	Unassigned
59	Outpatient

Exhibit 5–5 Example of Hospital Departmental Costs Classified by Diagnoses, MDC, and DRG

Hospital Departmental Code	DRG	Description	Cost
18 INFECTIOUS DISEASES	415	O/R—INFECT/PARASITIC DIS	$4,000
18 INFECTIOUS DISEASES	416	SEPTICEMIA)17	10,000
18 INFECTIOUS DISEASES	417	SEPTICEMIA 0–17	20,000
18 INFECTIOUS DISEASES	418	POSTOP/POSTTRAUMA INFECT	2,000
18 INFECTIOUS DISEASES	419	FEVER—UKN ORIG) 17W/C	3,000
18 INFECTIOUS DISEASES	420	FEVER—UKN ORIG) 17W/OC	6,000
18 INFECTIOUS DISEASES	421	VIRAL ILLNESS)17	4,000
18 INFECTIOUS DISEASES	422	VIR ILL/FEVER UNK 0–17	1,000
18 INFECTIOUS DISEASES	423	OT/INFECT/PARASITIC DX	3,000

If revenues are grouped by care setting or by service line, as discussed in the previous chapter, then expenses should also be grouped by these categories. In that way, matching of revenues and expenses can readily occur. A more detailed discussion of care settings and service lines, with examples, was presented in the preceding chapter.

Programs

A program can be defined as a project that has its own objectives and its own program indicators. Within management's functions of planning, controlling, and decision making, the program must stand on its own. A program is often funded separately and for finite periods of time. For example, funds from a grant might fund a specific project for, sayfor example, three years. Often programs—especially those funded separately from the revenue stream of the main organization—have to arrange their expenses in a special format that is specified by the entity that provides the grant funds.

Program expenses should be grouped in such a way that they are distinguishable. Also, if such programs have been especially funded, the reporting of their expenses should not be commingled. An example of a program cost center is given in Exhibit 5–6. This cost center example has received special funds and must be reported separately, as shown.

Table 5–1 Example of Radiology Department Costs Classified by Procedure Code

Procedure Code	Procedure Description	Department Cost
557210	Ribs, Unilateral	$60,000
557230	Spine Cervical Routine	125,000
557280	Pelvis	33,000
557320	Limb—Shoulder	55,000
557360	Limb—Wrist	69,000
557400	Limb—Hip, Unilateral	42,000
557410	Limb—Hip, Bilateral	14,000
557430	Limb—Knee Only	62,000
	Total	$460,000

COST REPORTS AS INFLUENCERS OF EXPENSE FORMATS

Cost reports are required by both the Medicare program (Title XVIII) and the Medicaid program (Title XIX). Every provider participating in the program is re-

Exhibit 5–6 Program Cost Center: Southside Homless Intake Center

Program:	Southside Homeless Intake Center
Department:	Feeding Ministry
For the Month of:	January 2000
Raw Food	$14,050
Dietary Supplies	200
Paper Supplies	300
Minor Equipment	50
Consultant Dietician	50
Utilities	300
Telephone	50
Program Total	$15,000

Table 5–2 Selected Cost Report Forms

Type	Form
Hospital complex (includes all hospital-based facilities)	HCFA 2552
Skilled nursing facility	HCFA 2540
Home health agencies	HCFA 1728
Comprehensive outpatient rehabilitation facilities	HCFA 2088

quired to file an annual cost report. An array of providers who must file cost reports is illustrated in Table 5–2. The arrangement of expense headings on the cost reports has been consistent since the advent of such reports in 1966. Therefore, this standard and traditional arrangement has strongly influenced the arrangement of expenses in many health care information systems.

The cost report uses a method of cost finding. Its focus is what is called a cost center. The concept is not the same as the type of responsibility center "cost center" that has been discussed earlier in this chapter. Instead, the cost-finding "cost center" is, broadly speaking, a type of cost pool used in the cost-finding process. The primary purpose of the cost pool/cost center in cost finding is to assist in allocating overhead.

The central worksheets for cost finding are Worksheet A, Worksheet B, and Worksheet B-1. Worksheet A contains the basic trial balance of all expenses for the facility. (Trial balances are discussed in a preceding chapter.) The beginning trial balance is reflected in the first three columns:

[Column 1]   [Column 2]   [Column 3]
 "Salaries"   +   "Other"   =   "Total"
                (all other expenses)

The trial balance is grouped at the outset into cost center categories. The placement of these categories and their respective line items on the page stay constant throughout the flow of Worksheets A, B, and B-1. The cost centers are grouped into seven categories:

1. General service
2. Inpatient routine service
3. Ancillary service
4. Outpatient service
5. Other reimbursable
6. Special purpose
7. Nonreimbursable

The line items within these seven categories represent the long-lived traditional arrangement that has strongly influenced the arrangement of expenses in so many health care information systems.

INFORMATION CHECKPOINT

What Is Needed?	A report that shows expense in your organization.
Where Is It Found?	With your supervisor.
How Is It Used?	Examine the report to find various types of expenses; look for how the expense flow is handled on the report.
What Is Needed?	A report that groups expenses by some type of classification.
Where Is It Found?	With your supervisor or in the information services division.
How Is It Used?	Examine the report to discover the methods that are used for grouping. You will probably find that these groupings are used for performance measures. They can also be used for control and planning.

 KEY TERMS

Cost
Diagnoses
Expenses
Expired Costs
General Services Expenses
Support Services Expenses
Operations Expenses
Procedures
Unexpired Costs

 DISCUSSION QUESTIONS

1. Have you worked with cost centers in your duties? If so, how have you been exposed to them?
2. Have you had to manage from a cost center type of report? If so, how was it categorized?
3. Do you believe that grouping expenses by diagnoses and procedures (based on type of services provided) is better to use for control and planning than grouping expenses by care setting (based on location of service provided)?
4. If so, why?
5. What grouping of expenses do you believe your organization uses (traditional cost centers, diagnoses/procedures, care settings, other)?
6. From your perspective, would there be a better grouping possible? If so, why do you think it is not used?

CHAPTER 6

Cost Classifications

PROGRESS NOTES

After completing this chapter, you should be able to

1. Distinguish between direct and indirect costs.
2. Understand why the difference is important to management.
3. Understand the composition and purpose of responsibility centers.
4. Distinguish between product and period costs.

DISTINCTION BETWEEN DIRECT AND INDIRECT COSTS

Direct costs can be specifically associated with a particular unit or department or patient. The critical distinction for the manager is that the cost is directly attributable. Whatever the manager is responsible for—that is, the unit, the department, or the patient—is known as a *cost object*.

The somewhat vague definition of a cost object is any unit for which a separate cost measurement is desired. It might help the manager to think of *cost object* as *cost objective*

instead.[1] The important thing is that direct costs can be traced. Indirect costs, on the other hand, cannot be specifically associated with a particular cost object. The controller's office is an example of indirect cost. The controller's office is essential to the overall organization itself, but its cost is not specifically—directly—associated with providing health care services. The critical distinction for the manager is that indirect costs usually cannot be traced but instead must be allocated or apportioned in some manner.[2] Figure 6–1 illustrates the direct–indirect cost distinction.

To summarize, it is helpful to recognize that direct costs are incurred for the sole benefit of a particular operating unit—a department, for example. As a rule of thumb, if the answer to the following question is "yes," then the cost is a direct cost: "If the operating unit (such as a department) did not exist, would this cost not be in existence?"

Indirect costs, in contrast, are incurred for the overall operation and not for any one unit. Because they are shared, indirect costs are sometimes called *joint costs* or *common costs*. As a rule of thumb, if the answer to the following question is "yes," then the cost is an indirect cost: "Must this cost be allocated in order to be assigned to the unit (such as a department)?"

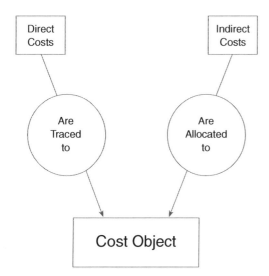

Figure 6–1 Assigning Costs to the Cost Object.

EXAMPLES OF DIRECT COST AND INDIRECT COST

It is important for managers to recognize direct and indirect costs and how they are treated on reports. Two sets of examples illustrate the reporting of direct and indirect costs. The first example concerns a radiology department; the second concerns a dialysis center.

Table 6–1 represents a report of two line items—direct costs and indirect costs—for a radiology department. The report concerns procedure numbers 557, 558, 559, 560, and 561 and a total. In this report, the manager can observe the proportionate differences between direct and indirect costs and can also see the differences among the five types of procedures.

Greater detail is provided to the manager in Table 6–2, which presents the method of allocating indirect costs and the result of such allocation. Managers should notice that the "totals" line carries forward and becomes the "indirect cost" line in Table 6–1. The purpose of the report in Table 6–2 is to reveal details that support the main report in Table 6–1. Thus, this report showing allocation of indirect costs is considered a subsidiary report because it is supporting, or subsidiary to, the preceding main report. This use of one or more supporting reports to reveal details behind the main report is quite common in managerial reports. The allocation of indirect costs subsidiary report contains quite a lot of information. It shows what line items (transporters, receptionists, etc.) are contained in the $1,267,000 total. It shows how each line item is allocated across the five separate procedures. And it

Table 6–1 Example of Radiology Departments Direct and Indirect Cost Totals

Dept: Radiology—Diagnostic
Cost Summary—Year to Date November 1999

Indirect Cost Centers	CC #557 Diagnostic Radiology	CC #558 Ultra- sound	CC #559 Nuclear Medicine	CC #560 CT Scan	CC #561 Radiation Therapy	Total
Direct costs	$1,000,000	$600,000	$1,200,000	$1,800,000	$1,400,000	$6,000,000
Indirect costs*	300,000	195,375	221,500	338,500	211,625	1,267,000
Totals	$1,300,000	$795,375	$1,421,500	$2,138,500	$1,611,625	$7,267,000

*See Table 6–2 for cost allocation detail.

Source: Adapted from A. Baptist, A General Approach to Costing Procedures in Ancillary Departments, *Topics in Health Care Financing,* Vol. 13, No. 4, p. 36, © 1987, Aspen Publishers, Inc.

Table 6–2 Example of Indirect Costs Allocated to Radiology Departments

Dept: Radiology—Diagnostic
Cost Summary—Year to Date November 1999

Indirect Cost Centers	Total Indirect Costs	Allocation Basis	CC #557 Diagnostic Radiology	CC #558 Ultrasound	CC #559 Nuclear Medicine	CC #560 CT Scan	CC #561 Radiation Therapy	Total
Transporters	$550,000	A	$110,000	$132,000	$88,000	$154,000	$66,000	$550,000
Receptionists	360,000	B	60,000	36,000	72,000	108,000	84,000	360,000
File room clerks	117,000	C	90,000	3,375	13,500	4,500	5,625	117,000
Managers	240,000	B	40,000	24,000	48,000	72,000	56,000	240,000
Totals	$1,267,000		$300,000	$195,375	$221,500	$338,500	$211,625	$1,267,000
Allocation Basis:								
A. Volumes			100,000	120,000	80,000	140,000	60,000	500,000
B. Direct costs			$1,000,000	$600,000	$1,200,000	$1,800,000	$1,400,000	$6,000,000
C. Number of films			400,000	15,000	60,000	20,000	25,000	520,000

Source: Adapted from A. Baptist, A General Approach to Costing Procedures in Ancillary Departments, *Topics in Health Care Financing,* Vol. 13, No. 4, p. 36, © 1987, Aspen Publishers, Inc.

shows how each line item was allocated; see the "Allocation Basis" column containing codes of A, B, C, and D. Then see the box below with the allocation basis set out for type (volumes/direct costs/number of films) and for resulting allocation of each across the five procedures. This set of tables is worthy of further study by the manager.

Exhibit 6–1 sets out the direct costs for a freestanding dialysis center. These costs, as direct costs, are what the organization's managers believe can be traced to the specific operation of the freestanding center. Exhibit 6–2 sets out the indirect costs for a freestanding dialysis center. These costs are what the organization's managers believe are not directly attributable to the specific operation of the freestanding center. The

Exhibit 6–2 Example of Freestanding Dialysis Center Indirect Costs

Indirect Costs	
Facility costs	$300,000
Administrative costs	300,000
Total indirect costs	$600,000

Courtesy of Resource Group, Ltd., Dallas, Texas.

decisions about what will and what will not be considered direct or indirect costs will almost always have been made for the manager.[3] What is important is that the manager understand two things: first, why this is so, and second, how the relationship between the two works. Remember the rule of thumb discussed earlier in this chapter. If the answer to the following question is "yes," then the cost is a direct cost: "If the operating unit (such as a department) did not exist, would this cost not be in existence?"

RESPONSIBILITY CENTERS

In a previous chapter, we discussed revenue centers, whereby managers are responsible for generating revenue (or volume). We also previously discussed cost centers, whereby managers are responsible for managing and controlling cost. The responsibility center makes a manager responsible for both the revenue/volume (inflow) side and the expense (outflow) side of a department, division, unit, or program. In other words, the manager is responsible for generating revenue/volume and for controlling costs. Another term for responsibility center is *profit center.*

We will examine the type of information a manager receives about his or her own responsibility center by reviewing the Westside

Exhibit 6–1 Example of Freestanding Dialysis Center Direct Costs

Salaries and fringe benefits	$500,000
Salaries—other professional	40,000
Medical director	40,000
Medical supplies	550,000
Pharmacy	1,130,000
Dialysis center equipment depreciation	80,000
Utilities	80,000
Housekeeping and laundry	20,000
Property taxes	40,000
Other supplies and costs	20,000
Total direct costs	$2,500,000

Source: Adapted from D.A. West, T.D. West, and P.J. Malone, Managing Capital and Administrative (Indirect) Costs to Achieve Strategic Objectives: The Dialysis Clinic versus the Outpatient Clinic, *Journal of Health Care Finance,* Vol. 25, No. 2, p. 24, © 1998, Aspen Publishers, Inc.

Center operations. Westside Center offers two basic types of services: an ambulatory surgery center and a rehabilitation center. The management of Westside is overseen by Bill, the director. Joe manages the ambulatory surgery center. Bonnie manages the rehabilitation center. Denise, a part-time radiologist, provides radiology services on an as-needed basis. Joe, Bonnie, and Denise, the managers, all report to Bill, the director. Figure 6–2 illustrates the managerial relationships.

To restate the relationships shown in Figure 6–2, Joe manages a responsibility center for ambulatory surgery services. Bonnie manages a responsibility center for rehabilitation services. These services represent the business of Westside Center. Denise manages the radiology services, but this is not a responsibility center in the Westside organization. Instead, it is a support center. Bill, the director, manages a bigger responsibility center that includes all of the functions just described plus the general and administrative support center.

Bill, the director, receives a managerial report shown in Exhibit 6–3. Bill's Director's Summary contains the data for the entire Westside operation.

Exhibit 6–3 Director's Summary of Westside ASC and Rehab Responsibility Center

ASC R/C Surplus	$70,000.00
Rehab R/C Surplus	85,000.00
Less G&A Support Ctr	(80,000.00)
Less Radiology Support Ctr	(20,000.00)
Net Surplus	$55,000.00

Courtesy of Resource Group, Ltd., Dallas, Texas.

Figure 6–3 illustrates the reports received by each manager at Westside. Joe's report for the ambulatory surgery center is at the top right of Figure 6–3. His report shows the controllable revenues he is responsible for ($225,000), less the controllable expenses he is responsible for ($150,000). The difference is labeled "ASC Responsibility Center Surplus" on his report. The surplus amounts to $70,000 ($225,000 minus $150,000).

Bonnie's report for the rehabilitation center is the second report on the right of Figure 6–3. Her report shows the controllable revenues she is responsible for ($300,000), less the controllable expenses she is respon-

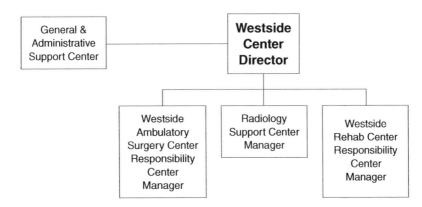

Figure 6–2 Lines of Managerial Responsibility at Westside Center. Courtesy of Resource Group, Ltd., Dallas, Texas.

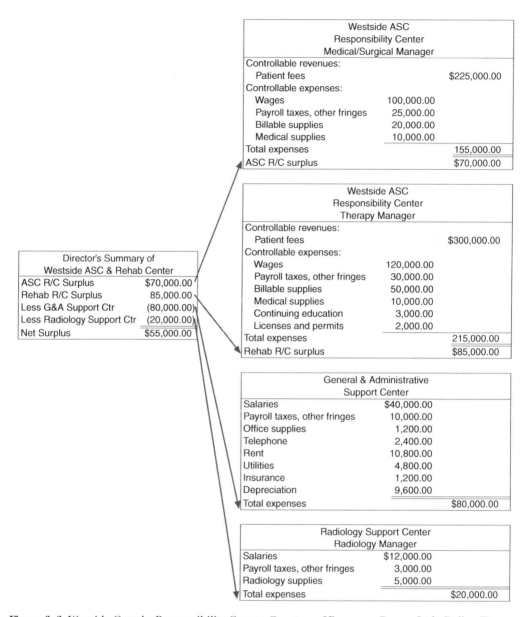

Figure 6–3 Westside Costs by Responsibility Center. Courtesy of Resource Group, Ltd., Dallas, Texas.

sible for ($215,000). The difference is labeled "Rehab Responsibility Center Surplus" on her report. The surplus amounts to $85,000 ($300,000 minus $215,000).

Denise's report for radiology services is at the bottom right of Figure 6–3. Her report shows the controllable expenses she is responsible for, which amount to $20,000. Her report shows only expenses because it is a support center, not a responsibility center. Therefore, Denise is responsible for expenses but not for revenue/volume.

Bill, the director, receives a report for the general and administrative (G&A) expenses, as shown second from the bottom right of Figure 6–3. This report shows the G&A controllable expenses that Bill himself is responsible for at Westside, which amount to $80,000. The G&A report shows only expenses because it also is a support center, not a responsibility center. Therefore, Bill is responsible for expenses but not for revenue/volume in the case of G&A.

However, Bill is also responsible for the entire Westside operation. That is, the overall Westside operation is his responsibility center. Therefore, Bill's Director's Summary, reproduced on the left side of Figure 6–3, contains the results of both responsibility centers and both support centers. The surplus figures from Joe and Bonnie's reports are positive figures of $70,000 and $85,000, respectively. The expense-only figures from Bill's G&A support center report and from Denise's radiology support center report are negative figures of $80,000 and $20,000, respectively. Therefore, to find the result of operations for Bill's entire Westside operation, the $80,000 and the $20,000 expense figures are subtracted from the surplus figures to arrive at a net surplus for Westside of $55,000.

Although the lines of managerial responsibility will vary in other organizations, the relationships between and among responsibility centers, support centers, and overall supervision will remain as shown in this example.

DISTINCTION BETWEEN PRODUCT AND PERIOD COSTS

Product costs is a term that was originally associated with manufacturing rather than with services. The concept of product costs assumes that a product has been manufactured and placed into inventory while waiting to be sold. Then, whenever that product is sold, the product is matched with revenue and recognized as a cost. Thus *cost of sales* is the common usage for manufacturing firms. (The concept of matching revenues and expenses has been discussed in a preceding chapter.)

Period costs, in the original manufacturing interpretation, are not connected with the manufacturing process. They are matched with revenue on the basis of the period during which the cost is incurred (thus *period costs*). The term comes from the span of time in which matching occurs, known as *time period*.

Service organizations have no manufacturing process as such. The business of health care service organizations is service delivery, not the manufacturing of products. Although the overall concept of product versus period cost is not as vital to service delivery, the distinction remains important for managers in health care to know.

In health care organizations, product cost can be viewed as traceable to the cost object of the department, division, or unit. A period cost is not traceable in this manner. Another way to view this distinction is to think of product costs as those costs necessary to actually deliver the service, whereas period costs are costs necessary to support the existence of the organization itself.

Finally, medical supply and pharmacy departments do have inventories on hand. In their case, a product is purchased (rather than manufactured) and placed into inventory while waiting to be dispensed. Then, whenever that product is dispensed, the product is matched with revenue and recognized as a cost of providing the service to the patient. Therefore, the product cost concept is important to managers of departments that hold a significant amount of inventory.

INFORMATION CHECKPOINT

What Is Needed?   Example of a management report that uses direct/indirect cost.

Where Is It Found?   With your supervisor, in administration, or in information services.

How Is It Used?   To track operations directly associated with the unit.

What Is Needed?   Example of a management report that uses responsibility centers.

Where Is It Found?   With your supervisor, in administration, or in information services.

How Is It Used?   To reflect operations that a manager is specifically responsible for and to measure those operations for planning and control.

 KEY TERMS

Cost Object
Direct Cost
Indirect Cost
Joint Cost
Responsibility Centers

 DISCUSSION QUESTIONS

1. In your own workplace, can you give a good example of a direct cost? An indirect cost?
2. What is the difference?
3. Does your organization use responsibility centers?
4. If not, do you think they should? Why?
5. If so, do you believe the responsibility centers operate properly? Would you make changes? Why?

PART III

Tools to Analyze Financial Operations

CHAPTER 7

Cost Behavior and Break-Even Analysis

PROGRESS NOTES

After completing this chapter, you should be able to

1. Understand the distinction between fixed, variable, and semivariable costs.
2. Be able to analyze mixed costs by two methods.
3. Understand the computation of a contribution margin.
4. Be able to compute the cost-volume-profit (CVP) ratio.
5. Be able to compute the profit-volume (PV) ratio.

DISTINCTION BETWEEN FIXED, VARIABLE, AND SEMIVARIABLE COSTS

This chapter emphasizes the distinction between fixed, variable, and semivariable costs because this knowledge is a basic working tool in financial management. The manager needs to know the difference between fixed and variable costs to compute contribution margins and break-even points. The manager also needs to know about semivariable costs to make good decisions about how to treat these costs.

Fixed costs are costs that do not vary in total when activity levels (or volume) of operations change. This concept is illustrated in Figure 7–1. The horizontal axis of the graph shows number of residents in the Jones Group Home, and the vertical axis shows total monthly fixed cost in dollars. In this graph, the total monthly fixed cost for the group home is $3,000, and that amount does not change, whether the number of residents (the activity level or volume) is low or high. A good example of a fixed cost is rent expense. Rent would not vary whether the home was almost full or almost empty; thus, rent is a fixed cost.

Variable costs, on the other hand, are costs that vary in direct proportion to changes in activity levels (or volume) of operations. This concept is illustrated in Figure 7–2. The horizontal axis of the graph shows number of residents in the Jones Group Home, and the vertical axis shows total monthly variable cost in dollars. In this graph, the monthly variable cost for the group home changes proportionately with the number of residents (the activity level or volume) in the home. A good example of a variable cost is food for the group home residents. Food would vary directly depending on the number of individuals in residence; thus, food is a variable cost.

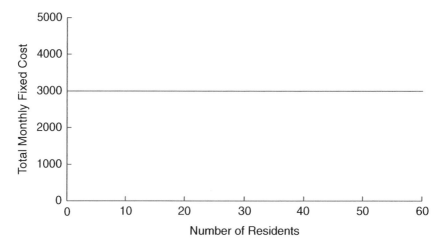

Figure 7–1 Fixed Costs—Jones Group Home.

Semivariable costs vary when the activity levels (or volume) of operations change, but not in direct proportion. The most frequent pattern of semivariable costs is the step pattern, where the semivariable cost rises, flattens out for a bit, and then rises again. The step pattern of semivariable costs is illustrated in Figure 7–3. The horizontal axis of the graph shows number of residents in the Jones Group Home, and the vertical axis shows total monthly semivariable cost. In this graph, the behavior of the cost line resembles stair steps: thus, the "step pattern" name for this configuration. The most common example of a semivariable expense in health care is supervisors' salaries. A single supervisor, for example, can perform adequately over a range of rises in activity levels (or volume). When another supervisor has to be added, the rise in the step pattern occurs.

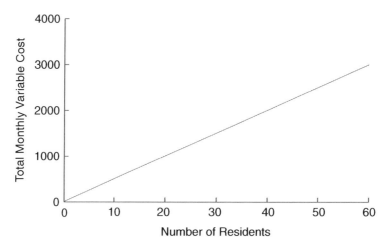

Figure 7–2 Variable Cost—Jones Group Home.

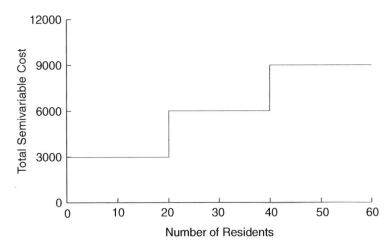

Figure 7–3 Semivariable Cost—Jones Group Home.

It is important to know, however, that there are two ways to think about fixed cost. The usual view is the flat line illustrated on the graph in Figure 7–1. That flat line represents total monthly cost for the group home. However, another perception is presented in Figure 7–4. The top view of fixed costs in Figure 7–4 is the usual flat line just discussed. The bottom view is fixed cost per resident. Think about the figure for a moment: the top view is dollars in total for the home for the month, and the bottom view is fixed-cost dollars by number of residents. The line is no longer flat but declines because this view of cost declines with each additional resident.

We can also think about variable cost in two ways. The usual view of variable cost is the diagonal line rising from the bottom of the graph to the top, as illustrated in Figure 7–2. That steep diagonal line represents monthly cost varying in direct proportion with number of residents in the home. However, another perception is presented in Figure 7–5. The top view of variable costs in Figure 7–5 represents total monthly variable cost and is the usual diagonal line just dis-

cussed. The bottom view is variable cost per resident. Think about this figure for a moment: the top view is dollars in total for the home for the month, and the bottom view is variable-cost dollars by number of residents. The line is no longer diagonal but is now flat because this view of variable cost stays the same proportionately for each resident. A good way to think about Figures 7–4 and 7–5 is to realize that they are close to being mirror images of each other.

Semifixed costs are sometimes used in health care organizations, especially in regard to staffing. Semifixed costs are the reverse of semivariable costs: that is, they stay fixed for a time as activity levels (or volume) of operations change, but then they will rise; then they will plateau; then they will rise. Thus, semifixed costs can exhibit a step pattern similar to that of variable costs.[1] However, the semifixed cost "steps" tend to be longer between rises in cost. In summary, both semifixed and semivariable costs have mixed elements of fixed and variable costs. Thus, both semivariable and semifixed costs are called *mixed costs.*

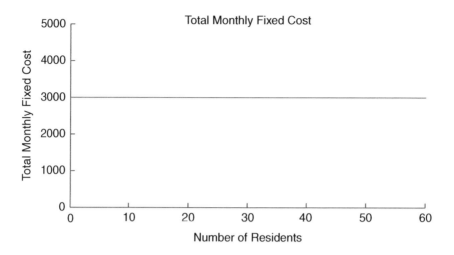

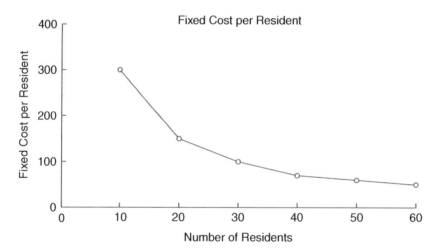

Figure 7–4 Two Views of Fixed Costs.

EXAMPLES OF VARIABLE AND FIXED COSTS

Studying examples of expenses that are designated as variable and fixed helps to understand the differences between them. It should also be mentioned that some expenses can be variable to one organization and fixed to another because they are handled differently by the two organizations. Operating room fixed and variable costs are illustrated in Table 7–1. Thirty-two expense accounts are listed in Table 7–1: 11 are variable, 20 are designated as fixed by this hospital, and 1, equipment depreciation, is listed separately.[2] (The separate listing is because of the way this hospital's accounting system handles equipment depreciation.)

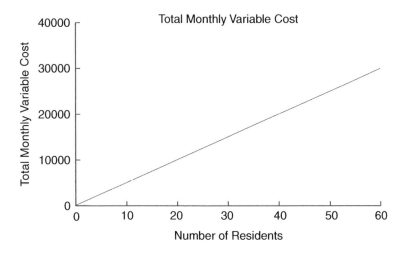

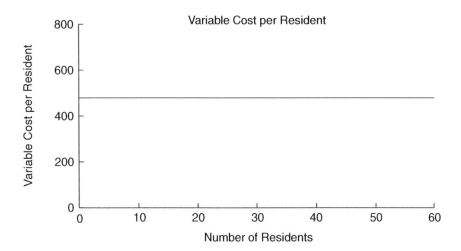

Figure 7–5 Two Views of Variable Costs.

Another example of semivariable and fixed staffing is presented in Table 7–2. The costs are expressed as full-time equivalent staff (FTEs). Each line-item FTE will be multiplied times the appropriate wage or salary to obtain the semivariable and fixed costs for the operating room. (The further use of FTEs for staffing purposes is fully discussed in the next chapter.) The supervisor position is fixed, which indicates that this is the minimum staffing that can be allowed. The single aide/orderly and the clerical position are also indicated as fixed. All the other positions—technicians, RNs, and LPNs—are listed as semivariable, which indicates that they are probably used in the semivariable

Table 7–1 Operating Room Fixed and Variable Costs

Account	Total	Variable	Fixed	Equipment
Social Security	$ 60,517	$ 60,517	$	$
Pension	20,675	20,675		
Health Insurance	8,422	8,422		
Child Care	4,564	4,564		
Patient Accounting	155,356	155,356		
Admitting	110,254	110,254		
Medical Records	91,718	91,718		
Dietary	27,526	27,526		
Medical Waste	2,377	2,377		
Sterile Procedures	78,720	78,720		
Laundry	40,693	40,693		
Depreciation—Equipment	87,378			87,378
Depreciation—Building	41,377		41,377	
Amortization—Interest	(5,819)		(5,819)	
Insurance	4,216		4,216	
Administration	57,966		57,966	
Medical Staff	1,722		1,722	
Community Relations	49,813		49,813	
Materials Management	64,573		64,573	
Human Resources	31,066		31,066	
Nursing Administration	82,471		82,471	
Data Processing	17,815		17,815	
Fiscal	17,700		17,700	
Telephone	2,839		2,839	
Utilities	26,406		26,406	
Plant	77,597		77,597	
Environmental Services	32,874		32,874	
Safety	2,016		2,016	
Quality Management	10,016		10,016	
Medical Staff	9,444		9,444	
Continuous Quality Improvement	4,895		4,895	
EE Health	569		569	
Total Allocated	$1,217,756	$600,822	$529,556	$87,378

Source: Adapted from J.J. Baker, *Activity-Based Costing and Activity-Based Management for Health Care*, p. 191, © 1998, Aspen Publishers, Inc.

step pattern that has been previously discussed in this chapter. This table is a good example of how to show clearly which costs will be designated as semivariable and which costs will be designated as fixed.

Another example illustrates the behavior of a single variable cost in a doctor's office. In Table 7–3, we see an array of costs for the procedure code 99214 office visit type. Nine costs are listed. The first cost is variable and is discussed momentarily. The other eight costs are all shown at the same level for a

Table 7–2 Operating Room Semivariable and Fixed Staffing

Job Positions	Total No. of FTEs	Semivariable	Fixed
Supervisor	2.2		2.2
Techs	3.0	3.0	
RNs	7.7	7.7	
LPNs	1.2	1.2	
Aides, orderlies	1.0		1.0
Clerical	1.2		1.2
Totals	16.3	11.9	4.4

99214 office visit: supplies, for example, is the same amount in all four columns. The single figure that varies is the top line, which is "report," meaning laboratory reports. This cost directly varies with the proportion of activity or volume, as variable cost has been defined. Here we see a variable cost at work: the first column on the left has no lab report, and the cost is zero; the second column has one lab report, and the cost is $3.82; the third column has two lab reports, and the cost is $7.64; and the fourth column has three lab reports, and the cost is $11.46.

The total cost rises by the same proportionate increase as the increase in the first line.

ANALYZING MIXED COSTS

It is important for planning purposes for the manager to know how to deal with mixed costs because they occur so often. For example, telephone, maintenance, repairs, and utilities are all actually mixed costs. The fixed portion of the cost is that portion representing having the service (such as telephone) ready to use, and the variable portion of the cost represents a portion of the charge for actual consumption of the service. We briefly discuss two very simple methods of analyzing mixed costs. Then we examine the high–low method and the scatter graph method.

Predominant Characteristics and Step Methods

Both the predominant characteristics and the step method of analyzing mixed costs are quite simple. In the predominant characteristic method, the manager judges whether the cost is more fixed or more

Table 7–3 Office Visit with Variable Cost of Tests

Service Code	99214 No Test	99214 1 Test	99214 2 Tests	99214 3 Tests
Report of lab tests	0.00	3.82	7.64	11.46
Fixed overhead	$31.00	$31.00	$31.00	$31.00
Physician	11.36	11.36	11.36	11.36
Medical assistant	1.43	1.43	1.43	1.43
Bill	0.45	0.45	0.45	0.45
Checkout	1.00	1.00	1.00	1.00
Receptionist	1.28	1.28	1.28	1.28
Collection	0.91	0.91	0.91	0.91
Supplies	0.31	0.31	0.31	0.31
Total visit cost	$47.74	$51.56	$55.38	$59.20

variable and acts on that judgment. In the step method, the manager examines the "steps" in the step pattern of mixed cost and decides whether the cost appears to be more fixed or more variable. Both methods are subjective.

High–Low Method

As the term implies, the high–low method of analyzing mixed costs requires that the cost be examined at its high level and at its low level. To compute the amount of variable cost involved, the difference in cost between high and low levels is obtained and is divided by the amount of change in the activity (or volume). Two examples are examined.

The first example is for an employee cafeteria. Table 7–4 contains the basic data required for the high–low computation. With the formula described in the preceding paragraph, the following steps are performed:

1. Find the highest volume of 45,000 meals at a cost of $165,000 in September (see Table 7–4) and the lowest volume of 20,000 meals at a cost of $95,000 in March.

2. Compute the variable rate per meal as

	No. of Meals	Employee Cafeteria Cost
Highest volume	45,000	$165,000
Lowest volume	20,000	95,000
Difference	25,000	70,000

3. Divide the difference in cost ($70,000) by the difference in number of meals (25,000) to arrive at the variable cost rate:

$70,000 divided by 25,000 meals =
$2.80 per meal

Table 7–4 Employee Cafeteria Number of Meals and Cost by Month

Month	No. of Meals	Employee Cafeteria Cost ($)
July	40,000	164,000
August	43,000	167,000
September	45,000	165,000
October	41,000	162,000
November	37,000	164,000
December	33,000	146,000
January	28,000	123,000
February	22,000	91,800
March	20,000	85,000
April	25,000	106,800
May	30,000	130,200
June	35,000	153,000

4. Compute the fixed overhead rate as follows:
   a. At the highest level:

Total cost	$165,000
Less: variable portion	
[45,000 meals × $2.80 @]	(126,000)
Fixed portion of cost	$39,000

   b. At the lowest level

Total cost	$95,000
Less: variable portion	
[20,000 meals × $2.80 @]	(56,000)
Fixed portion of cost	$39,000

   c. Proof totals: $39,000 fixed portion at both levels

The manager should recognize that large or small dollar amounts can be adapted to this method. A second example concerns drug samples and their cost. In this example, a supervisor of marketing is concerned about the number of drug samples used by the various members of the marketing staff. She uses the high–low method to determine the portion of fixed cost. Table 7–5 contains the basic data required for the high–low computation. Using the formula previously described, the following steps are performed:

1. Find the highest volume of 1,000 samples at a cost of $5,000 (see Table 7–5) and the lowest volume of 750 samples at a cost of $4,200.

2. Compute the variable rate per sample as

	No. of Samples	Cost
Highest volume	1,000	$5,000
Lowest volume	750	4,200
Difference	250	$800

3. Divide the difference in cost ($800) by the difference in number of samples (250) to arrive at the variable cost rate:

$800 divided by 250 samples = $3.20 per sample

4. Compute the fixed overhead rate as follows:
   a. At the highest level:

Total cost	$5,000
Less: variable portion [1,000 samples × $3.20 @]	(3,200)
Fixed portion of cost	$1,800

   b. At the lowest level

Total cost	$4,200
Less: variable portion [750 samples × $3.20 @]	(2,400)
Fixed portion of cost	$1,800

   c. Proof totals: $1,800 fixed portion at both levels

The high–low method is an approximation that is based on the relationship between the highest and the lowest levels, and the computation assumes a straight-line relationship. The advantage of this method is its convenience in the computation method.

Table 7–5 Number of Drug Samples and Cost for November

Rep.	No. of Samples	Cost
J. Smith	1,000	5,000
A. Jones	900	4,300
B. Baker	850	4,600
G. Black	975	4,500
T. Potter	875	4,750
D. Conner	750	4,200

CONTRIBUTION MARGIN, COST-VOLUME-PROFIT, AND PROFIT-VOLUME RATIOS

The manager should know how to analyze the relationship of cost, volume, and profit. This important information assists the manager in properly understanding and controlling operations. The first step in such analysis is the computation of the contribution margin.

Contribution Margin

The contribution margin is calculated in this way:

		% of Revenue
Revenues (net)	$500,000	100%
Less: variable cost	(350,000)	70%
Contribution margin	$150,000	30%
Less: fixed cost	(120,000)	
Operating income	$30,000	

The contribution margin of $150,000 or 30 percent in this example represents variable cost deducted from net revenues. The answer represents the contribution margin, so called because it contributes to fixed costs and to profits.

The importance of dividing costs into

fixed and variable becomes apparent now, for a contribution margin computation demands either fixed or variable cost classifications; no mixed costs are recognized in this calculation.

Cost-Volume-Profit (CVP) Ratio or Break Even

The break-even point is the point when the contribution margin (i.e., net revenues less variable costs) equals the fixed costs. When operations exceeds this break-even point, an excess of revenues over expenses (income) is realized. But if operations does not reach the break-even point, there will be an excess of expenses over revenues, and a loss will be realized.

The manager must recognize there are two ways of expressing the break-even point: either by an amount per unit or as a percentage of net revenues. If the contribution margin is expressed as a percentage of net revenues, it is often called the profit-volume (PV) ratio. A PV ratio example follows this cost-volume-profit (CVP) computation.

The CVP example is given in Figure 7–6. The data points for the chart come from the contribution margin as already computed:

		% of Revenue
Revenues (net)	$500,000	100%
Less: variable cost	(350,000)	70%
Contribution margin	$150,000	30%
Less: fixed cost	(120,000)	
Operating income	$30,000	

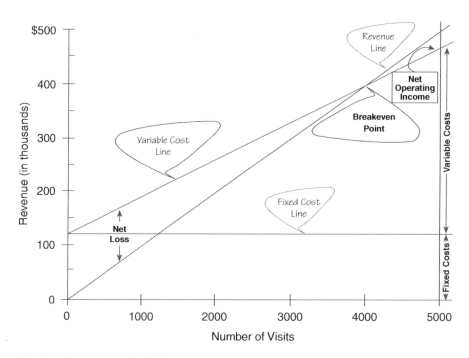

Figure 7–6 Cost-Volume-Profit (CVP) Chart for a Wellness Clinic. Courtesy of Resource Group, Ltd., Dallas, Texas.

Three lines were first drawn to create the chart. They were total fixed costs of $120,000, total revenue of $500,000, and variable costs of $350,000. (All three are labeled on the chart.) The break-even point appears at the point where the total cost line intersects the revenue line. Because this point is indeed the break-even point, the organization will have no profit and no loss but will break even. The wedge shape to the left of the break-even point is potential net loss, whereas the narrower wedge to the right is potential net income (both are labeled on the chart).

CVP charts allow a visual illustration of the relationships that are very effective for the manager.

Profit-Volume (PV) Ratio

Remember that the second method of expressing the break-even point is as a percentage of net revenues and that if the contribution margin is expressed as a percentage of net revenues, it is called the profit-volume (PV) ratio. Figure 7–7 illustrates the method. The basic data points used for the chart were as follows:

Revenue per visit	$100.00	100%
Less variable cost per visit	(70.00)	70%
Contribution margin per visit	$30.00	30%
Fixed costs per period	$120,000	

$30.00 contribution margin per visit divided by $100 price per visit = 30% PV Ratio

On our chart, the profit pattern is illustrated by a line drawn from the beginning level of fixed costs to be recovered ($120,000 in our case). Another line has been drawn straight across the chart at the break-even point. When the diagonal line begins at

$120,000, its intersection with the break-even or zero line is at $400,000 in revenue (see left-hand dotted line on chart). We can prove out the $120,000 versus $400,000 relationship as follows. Each dollar of revenue reduces the potential of loss by $0.30 (or 30 percent × $1.00). Fixed costs are fully recovered at a revenue level of $400,000, proved out as $120,000 divided by .30 = $400,000. This can be written as follows:

$$.30R = \$120,000$$
$$R = \$400,000 \ [120,000 \text{ divided by } .30 = 400,000].$$

The PV chart is very effective in planning meetings because only two lines are necessary to show the effect of changes in volume. Both PV and CVP are useful when working with the effects of changes in break-even points and revenue volume assumptions.

Contribution margins are also useful for showing profitability in other ways. An example appears in Figure 7–8, which shows the profitability of various DRGs, using contribution margins as the measure of profitability. Case volume (the number of cases of each DRG) is on the vertical axis of the matrix, and the dollar amount of contribution margin is on the horizontal axis of the matrix.

Scatter Graph Method

In performing a mixed-cost analysis, the manager is attempting to find the mixed cost's average rate of variability. The scatter graph method is more accurate than the high–low method previously described. It uses a graph to plot all points of data, rather than the highest and lowest figures used by the high–low method. Generally, cost will be on the vertical axis of the graph, and volume will be on the horizontal axis. All points are

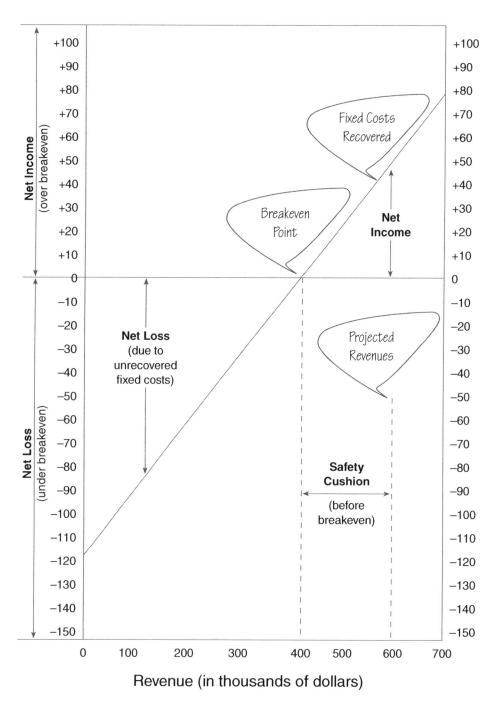

Figure 7–7 Profit-Volume (PV) Chart for a Wellness Clinic. Courtesy of Resource Group, Ltd., Dallas, Texas.

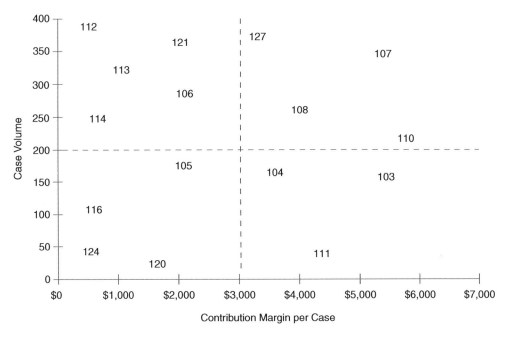

Figure 7–8 Profitability Matrix for Various DRGs, Using Contribution Margins. *Source:* Adapted from S. Upda, Activity-Based Costing for Hospitals, *Health Care Management Review,* Vol. 21, No. 3, p. 85, © 1996, Aspen Publishers, Inc.

plotted, each point being placed where cost and volume intersect for that line item. A regression line is then fitted to the plotted points. The regression line basically represents the average—or a line of averages. The average total fixed cost is found at the point where the regression line intersects with the cost axis.

Two examples are examined. They match the high–low examples previously calculated. Figure 7–9 presents the cafeteria data. The costs for cafeteria meals have been plotted on the graph, and the regression line has been fitted to the plotted data points. The regression line strikes the cost axis at a certain point; that amount represents the fixed cost portion of the mixed cost. The balance (or the total less the fixed cost portion) represents the variable portion.

The second example also matches the high–low example previously calculated. Figure 7–10 presents the drug sample data. The costs for drug samples have been plotted on the graph, and the regression line has been fitted to the plotted data points. The regression line again strikes the cost axis at the point representing the fixed-cost portion of the mixed cost. The balance (the total less the fixed cost portion) represents the variable portion. Further discussions of this method can be found in Exercises and Examples at the back of this book.

The examples presented here have regression lines fitted visually. However, com-

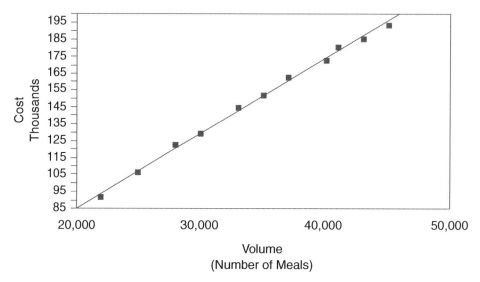

Figure 7–9 Employee Cafeteria Scatter Graph.

puter programs are available that will place the regression line through statistical analysis as a function of the program. This method is called the least-squares method. *Least squares* means that the sum of the squares of the deviations from plotted points to regression line is smaller than would occur from any other way the line could be fitted to the data: in other words, it is the best fit. This method is, of course, more accurate than fitting the regression line visually.

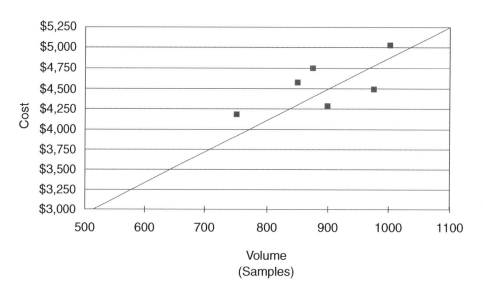

Figure 7–10 Drug Sample Scatter Graph for November.

INFORMATION CHECKPOINT

What Is Needed?	Revenues, variable cost, and fixed cost for a unit, division, DRG, etc.
Where Is It Found?	In operating reports.
How Is It Used?	Use the multiple-step calculations in this chapter to compute the CPV or the PV ratio; use to plan and control operations.

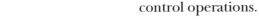 **KEY TERMS**

Break-even Analysis
Cost-Profit-Volume
Contribution margin
Fixed Cost
Mixed Cost
Profit-Volume Ratio
Semifixed Cost
Semivariable Cost
Variable Cost

 DISCUSSION QUESTIONS

1. Have you seen reports in your workplace that set out the contribution margin?
2. Do you believe that contribution margins can help you manage in your present work? In the future? How?
3. Have you encountered break-even analysis in your work?
4. If so, how was it used (or presented)?
5. How do you think you would use break-even analysis?
6. Do you believe your organization could use these analysis tools more often than is now happening? What do you believe the benefits would be?

CHAPTER 8

Staffing: The Manager's Responsibility

PROGRESS NOTES

After completing this chapter, you should be able to

1. Understand the difference between productive time and nonproductive time.
2. Understand computing full-time equivalents to annualize staff positions.
3. Understand computing full-time equivalents to fill a scheduled position.
4. Tie cost to staffing.

STAFFING REQUIREMENTS

In most businesses, a position is filled if the employee works five days a week, generally Monday through Friday. But in health care, many positions must be filled, or covered, all seven days of the week. Furthermore, in most businesses, a position is filled for that day if the employee works an eight-hour day—from 9:00 to 5:00, for example. But in health care, many positions must also be filled, or covered, 24 hours a day. The patients need care on Saturday and Sunday as well as Monday through Friday, and patients need care around the clock, 24 hours a day.

Thus, health care employees work in shifts. The shifts are often eight-hour shifts because three such shifts times eight hours apiece equals 24-hour coverage. Some facilities have gone to 12-hour shifts. In their case, two 12-hour shifts equal 24-hour coverage. The manager is responsible for seeing that an employee is present and working for each position and for every shift required for that position. Therefore, it is necessary to understand and use the staffing measurement known as the full-time equivalent (FTE). Two different approaches are used to compute FTEs: the annualizing method and the scheduled-position method. Full-time equivalent is a measure to express the equivalent of an employee (annualized) or a position (staffed) for the full time required. We examine both methods in this chapter.

FTEs FOR ANNUALIZING POSITIONS

Why Annualize?

Annualizing is necessary because each employee that is eligible for benefits (such as vacation days) will not be on duty for the full number of hours paid for by the organiza-

73

tion. Annualizing thus allows the full cost of the position to be computed through a "burden" approach. In the "burden" approach, the net hours desired are inflated, or burdened, in order to arrive at the gross number of paid hours that will be needed to obtain the desired number of net hours on duty from the employee.

Productive Versus Nonproductive Time

Productive time actually equates to the employee's net hours on duty when performing the functions in his or her job description. Nonproductive time is paid-for time when the employee is not on duty: that is, not producing and therefore "nonproductive." Paid-for vacation days, holidays, personal leave days, and/or sick days are all nonproductive time.[1]

Exhibit 8–1 illustrates productive time (net days when on duty) versus nonproductive time (additional days paid for but not worked). In Exhibit 8–1, Bob, the security guard, is paid for 260 days per year (total paid days) but works for only 235 days per year. The 235 days are productive time, and the remaining 25 days of holidays, sick days, vacation days, and education days are nonproductive time.

FTE for Annualizing Positions Defined

For purposes of annualizing positions, the definition of FTE is as follows: the equivalent of one full-time employee paid for one year, including both productive and nonproductive (vacation, sick, holiday, education, etc.) time. Two employees each working half-time for one year would be the same as one FTE.[1]

Staffing Calculations to Annualize Positions

Exhibit 8–2 contains a two-step process to perform the staffing calculation by the annualizing method. The first step computes the net paid days worked. In this step, the number of paid days per year is first arrived at; then paid days not worked are deducted to arrive at net paid days worked. The second step of the staffing calculation converts the net paid days worked to a factor. In the example in Exhibit 8–2, the factor averages out to about 1.6.

This calculation is for a 24-hour around-the-clock staffing schedule. Thus, the 364 in the step 2 formula equates to a 24-hour staffing expectation. Exhibit 8–3 illustrates such a master staffing plan.

NUMBER OF EMPLOYEES REQUIRED TO FILL A POSITION: ANOTHER WAY TO CALCULATE FTEs

Why Calculate by Position?

The calculation of number of FTEs by the schedule position method—in other words, to fill a position—is used in controlling, planning, and decision making. Exhibit 8–4 sets out the schedule and the FTE computation. A summarized explanation of the calculation in Exhibit 8–4 is as follows. One full-time employee (as shown) works 40 hours per week. One eight-hour shift per day times seven days per week equals 56 hours on duty. Therefore, to cover seven days per week or 56 hours requires 1.4 times a 40-hour employee (56 hours divided by 40 hours equals 1.4), or 1.4 FTEs.

Exhibit 8–1 Metropolis Clinic Security Guard Staffing

The Metropolis laboratory area has its own security guard from 8:30 AM to 4:30 PM seven days per week. Bob, the security guard for the clinic area, is a full-time Metropolis employee.
He works as follows:
1. The area assigned to Bob is covered seven days per week for every week of the year. Therefore,

Total days in business year	364
2. Bob doesn't work on weekends	(104)

(2 days per week × 52 weeks − 104 days)

Bob's paid days total per year amount to   260
(5 days per week × 52 weeks = 260 days)

3. During the year Bob gets paid for:

Holidays	9
Sick days	7
Vacation days	7
Education days	2

         (25)

4. Net paid days Bob actually works   235

Jim, a police officer, works part time as a security guard for the Metropolis laboratory area. Jim works on the days when Bob is off, including:

Weekends	104
Bob's holidays	9
Bob's sick days	7
Bob's vacation days	7
Bob's education days	2

         129

5. Paid days Jim works   129
6. Total days lab area security guard position is covered   364

Staffing Calculations to Fill Scheduled Positions

The term *staffing* as used here means the assigning of staff to fill scheduled positions. The staffing measure used to compute coverage is also called the FTE. It measures what proportion of one single full-time employee is required to equate the hours required (e.g., full time equivalent) for a particular position. For example, the cast room has to be staffed 24 hours a day seven days a week because it supports the emergency room and therefore has to provide service at any time. In this example, the employees are paid for an eight-hour shift. The three shifts

Exhibit 8–2 Basic Calculation for Annualizing Master Staffing Plan

Step 1: Compute Net Paid Days Worked

	RN	LPN	NA
Total Days in Business Year	364	364	364
Less Two Days off per Week	104*	104*	104*
No. of Paid Days per Year	260	260	260
Less Paid Days Not Worked:			
Holidays	9	9	9
Sick Days	7	7	7
Vacation Days	15	15	15
Education Days	3	2	1
Net Paid Days Worked	226	227	228

Step 2: Convert Net Paid Days Worked to a Factor

RN   Total days in business year divided by net paid days worked equals factor 364/226 = 1.6106195

LPN   Total days in business year divided by net paid days worked equals factor 364/227 = 1.6035242

NA   Total days in business year divided by net paid days worked equals factor 364/228 = 1.5964912

*Two days off per week equals $52 \times 2 = 104$.

Source: Data from J.J. Baker, *Prospective Payment for Long Term Care,* p. 116, © 1998, Aspen Publishers, Inc. and S.A. Finkler, *Budgeting Concepts for Nurse Managers,* 2nd ed., pp. 174–185, © 1992, W.B. Saunders Company.

Exhibit 8–3 Subacute Unit Master Staffing Plan

Staffing for Eight-Hour Nursing Shifts

	Shift 1 Day	+	Shift 2 Evening	+	Shift 3 Night	=	24-Hour Staff Total
RN	2		2		1		5
LPN	1		1		1		3
NA	5		4		2		11

Source: Adapted from J.J. Baker, *Prospective Payment for Long Term Care,* p. 116, © 1998, Aspen Publishers, Inc.

Exhibit 8–4 Staffing Requirements Example

Emergency Department Scheduling for Eight-Hour Shifts:				
	Shift 1 Day	Shift 2 Evening	Shift 3 Night	24-Hour Scheduling = Total
Position: Emergency Room Intake	1	1	1	= 3 8-hour shifts
To Cover Position Seven Days per Week Equals FTEs of:	1.4	1.4	1.4	= 4.2 FTEs

One full-time employee works 40 hours per week. One eight-hour shift per day times seven days per week equals 56 hours on duty. Therefore, to cover seven days per week or 56 hours requires 1.4 times a 40-hour employee (56 hours divided by 40 hours equals 1.4), or 1.4 FTEs.

required to fill the position for 24 hours are called the day shift (7:00 AM to 3:00 PM), the evening shift (3:00 PM to 11:00 PM), and the night shift (11:00 PM to 7:00 AM).

One eight-hour shift times five days per week equals a 40-hour work week. One 40-hour work week times 52 weeks equals a person-year of 2,080 hours. Therefore, one person-year of 2,080 hours equals a full-time position filled for one full year. This measure is our baseline.

It takes seven days to fill the day shift cast room position from Monday through Sunday, as required. Seven days is 140 percent of five days (seven divided by five equals 140 percent), or, expressed another way, is 1.4. The FTE for the day shift cast room position is 1.4. If a seven-day schedule is required, the FTE will be 1.4.

This method of computing FTEs uses a basic 40-hour work week (or 37-hour work week, or whatever is the case in the particular institution). The method computes a fig-

ure that will be necessary to fill the position for the desired length of time, measuring this figure against the standard basic work week. For example, if the standard work week is 40 hours and a receptionist position is to be filled for just 20 hours per week, then the FTE for that position would be 0.5 FTE (20 hours to fill the position divided by a 40-hour standard work week). Table 8–1 illustrates the difference between a standard work year at 40 hours per week and a standard work year at 37.5 hours per week.

TYING COST TO STAFFING

In the case of the annualizing method, the factor of 1.6 already has this organization's vacation, holiday, sick pay, and other nonproductive days accounted for in the formula (review Exhibit 8–2 to check out this fact). Therefore, this factor is multiplied times the base hourly rate (the net rate) paid to compute cost.

Table 8–1 Calculations to Staff the Operating Room

Job Position	No. of FTEs	No. of Annual Hours Paid at 2,080 Hours*	No. of Annual Hours Paid at 1,950 Hours
Supervisor	2.2	4,576	4,290
Techs	3.0	6,240	5,850
RNs	7.7	16,016	15,015
LPNs	1.2	2,496	2,340
Aides, orderlies	1.0	2,080	1,950
Clerical	1.2	2,496	2,340
Totals	16.3	33,904	31,785

*40 hours per week × 52 weeks = 2,080.
37.5 hours per week × 52 weeks = 1,950.

In the case of the scheduled-position method, however, the FTE figure of 1.4 will be multiplied times a burdened hourly rate. The burden on the hourly rate reflects the vacation, holiday, sick pay, and other nonproductive days accounted for in the formula (review Exhibit 8–4 to see the difference). The scheduled-position method is often used in the forecasting of new programs and services.

Actual cost is attached to staffing in the books and records through a subsidiary journal and a basic transaction record (both discussed in a preceding chapter). Exhibit 8–5 illustrates a subsidiary journal in which employee hours worked for a one-week period are recorded. Both regular and overtime hours are noted. The hourly rate, base pay, and overtime premiums are noted, and gross earnings are computed. Deductions are noted and deducted from gross earnings to compute the net pay for each employee in the final column.

Exhibit 8–6 illustrates a time card for one employee for a week-long period. This type of record, whether it is generated by a time clock or an electronic entry, is the original

record upon which the payroll process is based. Thus, it is considered a basic transaction record. In this example, time in and time out are recorded daily. The resulting regular and overtime hours are recorded separately for each day worked. Although the appearance of the time card may vary, the essential transaction is the same: this recording of daily time is where the payroll process begins.

Exhibit 8–7 represents an emergency department staffing report. Actual productive time is shown in columns 1 and 2, with regular time in column 1 and overtime in column 2. Nonproductive time is shown in column 3, and columns 1, 2, and 3 are totaled to arrive at column 4, labeled "Total [actual] Hours." The final actual figure is the FTE figure in column 5.

The report is biweekly and thus is for a two-week period. The standard work week amounts to 40 hours, so the biweekly standard work period amounts to 80 hours. Note the first line item, which is for the manager of the emergency department nursing service. The actual hours worked in column 4 amount to 80, and the actual FTE

Exhibit 8–5 Example of a Payroll Register

Metropolis Health System
Payroll Register

Week Ended _____ June 10, 2000

Employee No.	Name	Hours Worked			Rate	Base Pay	Overtime Premiums	Gross Earnings	Deductions					Net Pay
		Regular	Overtime	Total					Federal Income Tax	Social Security	Medicare Tax			
1071	J.F. Green	40	2	42	14.00	588.00	14.00	602.00	90.30	37.32	8.73			465.65
1084	C.B. Brown	40		40	14.00	560.00		560.00	84.00	34.72	8.62			432.66
1090	K.D. Grey	40		40	10.00	400.00		400.00	60.00	24.80	6.16			309.04
1092	R.N. Black	40	5	45	10.00	450.00	25.00	475.00	71.25	29.45	6.89			367.41

Courtesy of Resource Group, Ltd., Dallas, Texas.

Exhibit 8–6 Example of a Time Record

Metropolis Health System
Time Card

Employee ___J.F. Green___   No. _____1071_____

Department _____3_____ Week ending _____June 10_____

Day	Regular				Overtime		Hours	
	In	Out	In	Out	In	Out	Regular	Overtime
Monday	8:00	12:01	1:02	5:04			8	
Tuesday	7:56	12:00	12:59	5:03	6:00	8:00	8	2
Wednesday	7:57	12:02	12:58	5:00			8	
Thursday	8:00	12:00	1:00	5:01			8	
Friday	7:59	12:01	1:01	5:02			8	
Saturday								
Sunday								
					Total regular hours		40	
					Total overtime			2

Courtesy of Resource Group, Ltd., Dallas, Texas.

figure in column 5 is 1.0. We can tell from this line item that the second method of computing FTEs—the FTE computation to fill scheduled positions—has been used in this case. Columns 7 through 9 report budgeted time and FTEs, and columns 10 through 12 report the variance in actual from budget. The budget and variance portions of this report will be more thoroughly discussed in Chapter 13.

In summary, hours worked and pay rates are essential ingredients of staffing plans, budgets, and forecasts. Appropriate staffing is the responsibility of the manager.

Exhibit 8–7 Comparative Hours Staffing Report

PR 2301

Biweekly Comparative Hours Report
For the Payroll Period Ending Sept. 20, 2000

Dept. No. 3421
Emergency Room

		Actual					Budget				Variance		
		Productive											
	Job Code	Regular Time (1)	Overtime (2)	Non-Productive (3)	Total Hours (4)	FTEs (5)	Productive (6)	Non-Productive (7)	Total Hours (8)	FTEs (9)	Number Hours (10)	Number FTEs (11)	Percent (12)
Mgr Nursing Service	11075	80	0	0	80	1.0	69.8	10.2	80	1	0	0	0
Supv Charge Nurse	11403	383.2	0.1	79	462.3	5.8	456	64	520	6.5	57.7	0.7	11.1%
Medical Assistant	12007	6.2	0	0	6.2	0.1	0	0	0	0	-6.2	-0.1	100.0%
Staff RN	13401	2010.5	32.8	285.8	2329.1	29.1	2012.8	240.8	2253.6	28.2	-75.5	-0.9	-3.4%
Relief Charge Nurse	13403	81.9	4.3	0	86.2	1.1	0	0	0	0	-86.2	-1.1	100.0%
Orderly/Transporter	15483	203.8	38	20	261.8	3.3	279.8	35.3	315.1	3.9	53.3	0.6	16.9%
ER Tech	22483	244.6	27.5	67.9	340	4.3	336.2	34.5	370.7	4.6	30.7	0.3	8.3%
Secretary	22730	58.1	0	0	58.1	0.7	50.5	5.9	56.4	0.7	-1.7	0.0	-3.0%
Unit Coordinator	22780	555.1	35.6	74.9	665.6	8.3	505.4	53.8	559.2	7	-106.4	-1.3	-19.0%
Preadmission Testing Clerk	22818	0	6.5	0	6.5	0.1	0	0	0	0	-6.5	-0.1	100.0%
Patient Registrar	22873	617.5	78.6	105.7	801.8	10.0	718.2	57.8	776	9.7	-25.8	-0.3	-3.3%
Lead Patient Registrar	22874	0	0	0	0	0.0	73.8	6.2	80	1	80.0	1.0	100.0%
Patient Registrar (weekend)	22876	36.7	0	0	36.7	0.5	0	0	0	0	-36.7	-0.5	100.0%
Overtime	29998	0	0	0	0	0.0	38.5	0	38.5	0.5	38.5	0.5	100.0%
Department Totals		4277.6	223.4	633.3	5134.3	64.3	4541	508.5	5049.5	63.1	-84.8	-1.2	0.0

Courtesy of Resource Group, Ltd., Dallas, Texas

INFORMATION CHECKPOINT

What Is Needed?   The original record of time and the subsidiary journal
                              summary.
Where Is It Found?   The original record can be found at any check-in point;
                              the subsidiary journal summary can be found with a
                              supervisor in charge of staffing for a unit, division,
                              etc.
How Is It Used?   It is reviewed as historical evidence of results achieved. It
                              is also reviewed by managers seeking to perform fu-
                              ture staffing in an efficient manner.

 KEY TERMS

Full-Time Equivalents (FTEs)
Nonproductive Time
Productive Time
Staffing

 DISCUSSION QUESTIONS

1. Are you or your immediate supervisor responsible for staffing?
2. If so, do you use a computerized program?
3. Do you believe a computerized program is better? If so, why?
4. Does your organization report time as "productive" and "nonproductive"?
5. If not, do you believe it should? What do you believe the benefits would be?

PART IV

Report and Measure Financial Results

CHAPTER 9

Reporting

PROGRESS NOTES

After completing this chapter, you should be able to

1. Review a balance sheet and understand its components.
2. Review a statement of revenue and expense and understand its components.
3. Understand the basic concept of cash flows.
4. Know what a subsidiary report is.

UNDERSTANDING THE MAJOR REPORTS

It is not our intention to convert you into an accountant. Therefore, our discussion of the major financial reports will center on the concept of each report and not on the precise accounting entries that are necessary to make the statement balance. The first concept we will discuss is that of cash versus accrual accounting. In cash basis accounting, a transaction does not enter the books until cash is either received or paid out. In accrual accounting, revenue is recorded when it is earned—not when payment is received—and expenses are recorded when they are incurred—not when they are paid.[1] Most health care organizations operate on the accrual basis.

There are four basic financial statements. You can think of them as a set. They include the balance sheet, the statement of revenue and expense, the statement of fund balance or net worth, and the statement of cash flows. The four major reports we are about to examine—the financial statements—have been prepared using the accrual method.

BALANCE SHEET

The balance sheet records what an organization owns, what it owes, and basically, what it is worth (although the terminology uses fund balance rather than worth or equity for nonprofit organizations). The balance sheet balances. That is, the total of what the organization owns—its assets—equals the combined total of what the organization owes and what it is worth—that is, its liabilities and its net worth or its fund balance. This balancing of the elements in the balance sheet can be visualized as

$$\text{Assets} = \text{Liabilities} + \text{Net Worth/Fund Balance}$$

Another characteristic of the balance sheet is that it is stated at a particular point in time. A common analogy is that a balance sheet is like a snapshot: it freezes the figures and reports them as of a certain date.

Exhibit 9–1 illustrates these concepts. A single date (not a period of time) is at the top of the statement (this is the snapshot). The clinic balance sheet reflects two years in two columns, with the most current date on

Exhibit 9–1 Westside Clinic Balance Sheet

Assets	December 31, 20x7		December 31, 20x8	
Currents Assets				
Cash and cash equivalents		$190,000		$145,000
Accounts receivable (net)		250,000		300,000
Inventories		25,000		20,000
Prepaid insurance		5,000		3,000
Total current assets		$470,000		$468,000
Property, Plant, and Equipment				
Land	$100,000		$100,000	
Buildings (net)	0		0	
Equipment (net)	260,000		300,000	
Net property, plant, and equipment		360,000		400,000
Other Assets				
Investments	$133,000		$32,000	
Total other assets		133,000		32,000
Total Assets		$963,000		$900,000
Liabilities and Fund Balance				
Current Liabilities				
Current maturities of long-term debt	$52,000		$48,000	
Accounts payable and accrued expenses	293,000		302,000	
Total current liabilities		$345,000		$350,000
Long-Term Debt	$252,000		$300,000	
Less Current Maturities of Long-Term Debt	(52,000)		(48,000)	
Net Long-Term Debt		200,000		252,000
Total liabilities		$545,000		$602,000
Fund Balances				
Unrestricted fund balance	$418,000		$298,000	
Restricted fund balance	0		0	
Total fund balances		418,000		298,000
Total Liabilities and Fund Balance		$963,000		$900,000

Courtesy of Resource Group, Ltd., Dallas, Texas.

the left and the prior period on the right. Total assets for the current left-hand column amount to $963,000. Total liabilities and fund balance also amount to $963,000; the balance sheet balances. The total liabilities amount to $545,000 and the total fund balances amount to $418,000. The total of the two, of course, makes up the $963,000 shown at the bottom of the statement.

Three types of assets are shown: current assets; property, plant, and equipment; and other assets. Current assets are supposed to be convertible into cash within one year—thus "current" assets. Property, plant, and equipment, however, represent long-term assets. Other assets represent noncurrent items.

Two types of liabilities are shown: current liabilities and long-term debt. Current liabilities are those expected to be paid within the next year—thus "current" liabilities. Long-term debt is not due within a year. (In fact, most long-term debt is due over a period of many years.) The amount of long-term debt that will be due within the next year ($52,000) has been subtracted from the long-term debt amount and has been moved up into the current liabilities section. This treatment is consistent with the concept of "current."

Because our intent is not to make an accountant of you, we will not be discussing generally accepted accounting principles (GAAPs) either. Financial accounting and the resulting reports intended for third-party use must be prepared in accordance with GAAPs. However, managerial accounting for internal purposes in the organization does not necessarily have to adhere to GAAPs. One of the requirements of GAAPs is that unrestricted fund balances be separated from restricted fund balances on the statements, so you see two appropriate line items (restricted and unrestricted) in the fund balance section.

STATEMENT OF REVENUE AND EXPENSE

The formula for a very condensed statement of revenue and expense would look like this:

Operating Revenue – Operating Expenses = Operating Income

A statement of revenue and expense covers a period of time (rather than one single date or point in time). The concept is that revenue, or inflow, less expenses, or outflow, results in an excess of revenue over expenses if the year has been good, or perhaps an excess of expenses over revenue (resulting in a loss) if the year has been bad.

Exhibit 9–2 sets out the result of operations for two years, with the most current period in the left columns. If the balance sheet is a snapshot, then the statement of revenue and expenses is a diary because it is a record of transactions over the period of a year. Operating revenues and operating expenses are set out first, with the result being income from operations of $115,000 ($2,000,000 less $1,885,000). Then other transactions are reported; in this case, interest income of $5,000 under the heading "Nonoperating Gains (Losses)." The total of $120,000 ($115,000 plus $5,000) is reported as an increase in fund balance. This figure carries forward to the next major report, known as the statement of changes in fund balance.

STATEMENT OF CHANGES IN FUND BALANCE/NET WORTH

Remember that our formula for a basic statement of revenue and expense looked like this:

Operating Revenue – Operating Expenses = Operating Income

Exhibit 9–2 Westside Clinic Statement of Revenue and Expenses

Revenue		December 31, 20x7		December 31, 20x8
Net patient service revenue		$2,000,000		$1,850,000
Total operating revenue		$2,000,000		$1,850,000
Operating Expenses				
Medical/surgical services	$600,000		$575,000	
Therapy services	860,000		806,000	
Other professional services	80,000		75,000	
Support services	220,000		220,000	
General services	65,000		60,000	
Depreciation	40,000		40,000	
Interest	20,000		24,000	
Total operating expenses		1,885,000		1,800,000
Income from Operations		$115,000		$50,000
Nonoperating Gains (Losses)				
Interest income	$5,000		$2,000	
Net nonoperating gains		5,000		2,000
Revenue and Gains in Excess of				
Expenses and Losses		$120,000		$52,000
Increase in Unrestricted Fund Balance		$120,000		$52,000

    Courtesy of Resource Group, Ltd., Dallas, Texas.

The excess of revenue over expenses flows back into equity or fund balance through the mechanism of the statement of fund balance/net worth. Exhibit 9–3 shows a balance at the first of the year; then it adds the excess of revenue over expenses (in the amount of $115,000) plus some interest income (in the amount of $5,000) to arrive at the balance at the end of the year.

If you refer back to the balance sheet, you will see the $418,000 balance at the end of the year appearing on it. So we can think of the balance sheet, the statement of revenue and expenses, and the statement of changes in fund balance/net worth as locked together, with the statement of changes in fund balance being the mechanism that links the other two statements.

But there is one more major report—the statement of cash flows—and we will examine it next.

STATEMENT OF CASH FLOWS

To perceive why a statement of cash flows is necessary, we must first revisit the concept of accrual basis accounting. If cash is not paid or received when revenues and expenses are entered on the books—the usual situation in accrual accounting—what happens? The other side of the entry for revenues is accounts receivable, and the other side of the entry for expenses is accounts payable. These accounts rest on the balance sheet and have not yet been turned into cash. Another characteristic of accrual accounting is

Exhibit 9–3 Westside Clinic Statement of Changes in Fund Balance

	For the Year Ending	
Statement of Changes in Fund Balance	December 31, 20x7	December 31, 20x8
Balance First of Year	$298,000	$246,000
Revenue in Excess of Expenses	115,000	50,000
Interest Income	5,000	2,000
Balance End of Year	$418,000	$298,000

Courtesy of Resource Group, Ltd., Dallas, Texas.

the recognition of depreciation. A capital asset—a piece of equipment, for example—is purchased for $20,000. It has a usable life of five years. So depreciation expense is recognized in each of the five years until the $20,000 is used up, or depreciated. Depreciation is recognized within each year as an expense, but it does not represent a cash expense. This is a concept that now enters into the statement of cash flows.

Exhibit 9–4 presents the current period cash flow. In effect, this statement takes the accrual basis statements and converts them to a cash flow for the period through a series of reconciling adjustments that account for the noncash amounts.

Understanding the cash/noncash concept makes sense of this statement. The starting point is the income from operations, the final item on the statement of revenue and expense. Depreciation and interest are added back, and changes in asset and liability accounts, both positive and negative, are recognized. These adjustments account for operating activities. Next, capital and related financing activities are addressed; then investing activities are adjusted. The result is a net increase in cash and cash equivalents of $45,000 in our example. This figure is added to the cash balance at the beginning of the

year ($145,000) to arrive at the cash balance at the end of the year ($190,000). Now refer back to the balance sheet, and you will find the cash balance is indeed $190,000. So the fourth major report—the statement of cash flows—interlocks with the other three major reports.

SUBSIDIARY REPORTS

The subsidiary reports are just that: subsidiary to the major reports. These reports support the major reports by providing more detail. For example, patient service revenue totals on the statement of revenue and expenses are often expanded in more detail on a subsidiary report. The same thing is true of operating expense. These reports are called "schedules" instead of "statements"—a sure sign that they are subsidiary reports.

SUMMARY

The four major reports fit together; each makes its own contribution to the whole. A checklist for balance sheet review (Exhibit 9–5) and a checklist for review of the statement of revenue and expense (Exhibit 9–6) are provided.

Exhibit 9–4 Westside Clinic Statement of Cash Flows

	For the Year Ending	
Statement of Cash Flows	December 31, 20x7	December 31, 20x8
Operating Activities		
Income from operations	$115,000	$50,000
Adjustments to reconcile income from operations to net cash flows from operating activities		
Depreciation and amortization	40,000	40,000
Interest expense	20,000	24,000
Changes in asset and liability accounts		
Patient accounts receivable	50,000	(250,000)
Inventories	(5,000)	(5,000)
Prepaid expenses and other assets	(2,000)	(1,000)
Accounts payable and accrued expenses	(9,000)	185,000
Net cash flow from operating activities	$209,000	$43,000
Cash Flows from Noncapital Financing Activities	0	0
Cash Flows from Capital and Related Financing Activities		
Acquisition of equipment	$0	$(300,000)
Proceeds from loan for equipment	0	300,000
Interest paid on long-term obligations	(20,000)	0
Repayment of long-term obligations	(48,000)	0
Net cash flows from capital and related financing activities	(68,000)	0
Cash Flows from Investing Activities		
Interest income received	$5,000	$2,000
Investments purchased (net)	(101,000)	0
Net cash flows from investing activities	(96,000)	2,000
Net Increase (Decrease) in Cash and Cash Equivalents	$45,000	$45,000
Cash and Cash Equivalents, Beginning of Year	145,000	100,000
Cash and Cash Equivalents, End of Year	$190,000	$145,000

Courtesy of Resource Group, Ltd., Dallas, Texas.

Exhibit 9–5 Checklist for Balance Sheet Review

1. What is the date on the balance sheet?
2. Are there large discrepancies in balances between the prior year and the current year?
3. Did total assets increase over the prior year?
4. Did current assets increase, decrease, or stay about the same?
5. Did current liabilities increase, decrease, or stay about the same?
6. Did land, plant, and equipment increase or decrease significantly over the prior year?
7. Did long-term debt increase or decrease significantly over the prior year?

Exhibit 9–6 Checklist for Review of the Statement of Revenue and Expense

1. What is the period reported on the statement of revenue and expense?
2. Is it one year or a shorter period? If it is a shorter period, why is that?
3. Are there large discrepancies in balances between the prior year operations and the current year operations?
4. Did total operating revenue increase over the prior year?
5. Did total operating expenses increase, decrease, or stay about the same? Is any particular line item unusually large or small?
6. Did income from operations increase, decrease, or stay about the same?
7. Are there unusual nonoperating gains or losses?
8. Did the current year result in an excess of revenue over expense? Is it as much as the prior year?
9. Did long-term debt increase or decrease significantly over the prior year?

 INFORMATION CHECKPOINT

What Is Needed?	A set of financial statements, ideally containing the four major reports plus subsidiary reports for additional detail.
Where Is It Found?	Possibly in the files of your supervisor or in the finance offices or in the office of the administrator.
How Is It Used?	Study the financial statement to see how they fit together; use the checklists included in this chapter to assist in your review. Understanding how the statements work will give you another valuable managerial tool.

KEY TERMS

Accrual Basis of Accounting
Balance Sheet
Cash Basis of Accounting
Statement of Revenue and Expense
Statement of Cash Flows
Statement of Fund Balance/Net Worth
Subsidiary Reports

 DISCUSSION QUESTIONS

1. Can you give an example of an asset? A liability?
2. Does the concept of revenue less expense equaling an increase in equity or fund balance make sense to you? If not, why not?
3. Are you familiar with the current maturity of long-term debt? What example of it can you give in your own life (either at work or at home)?
4. Do you get a chance to review financial statements at your place of work? Would you like to? Why?

CHAPTER 10

Financial and Operating Ratios as Performance Measures

After completing this chapter, you should be able to

1. Understand four types of liquidity ratios.
2. Understand two types of solvency ratios.
3. Understand two types of profitability ratios.
4. Successfully compute ratios.

THE IMPORTANCE OF RATIOS

Ratios are convenient and uniform measures that are widely adopted in health care financial management. They are important because they are so widely used, especially because they are used for credit analysis. But a ratio is only a number. It has to be considered within the context of the operation. There is another caveat: ratio analysis should be conducted as a comparative analysis. In other words, one ratio standing alone with nothing to compare it with does not mean very much. When interpreting ratios, the differences between periods must be considered, and the reasons for such differences should be sought. It is a good practice to compare results with equivalent computations from outside the organization—regional figures from similar institutions would be a good example of such outside sources. Caution and good managerial judgment must always be exercised when working with ratios.

Financial ratios basically pull together two elements of the financial statements: one expressed as the numerator and one as the denominator. To calculate a ratio, divide the bottom number (the denominator) into the top number (the numerator). Mini Case Study A in Chapter 19 uses financial ratios as indicators of financial position. We highly recommend that you spend time with this Mini Case Study, as it will add depth and background to the contents of this chapter.

In this chapter we examine liquidity, solvency, and profitability ratios. Exhibit 10–1 sets out eight basic ratios that are widely used in health care organizations: four liquidity types, two solvency types, and two profitability types. All are discussed later here.

LIQUIDITY RATIOS

Liquidity ratios reflect the ability of the organization to meet its current obligations.

Exhibit 10–1 Eight Basic Ratios Used in Health Care

Liquidity Ratios

1. Current Ratio

$$\frac{\text{Current Assets}}{\text{Current Liabilities}}$$

2. Quick Ratio

$$\frac{\text{Cash and Cash Equivalents} + \text{Net Receivables}}{\text{Current Liabilities}}$$

3. Days Cash on Hand (DCOH)

$$\frac{\text{Unrestricted Cash and Cash Equivalents}}{\text{Cash Operation Expenses} \div \text{No. of Days in Period (365)}}$$

4. Days Receivables

$$\frac{\text{Net Receivables}}{\text{Net Credit Revenues} \div \text{No. of Days in Period (365)}}$$

Solvency Ratios

5. Debt Service Coverage Ratio (DSCR)

$$\frac{\text{Change in Unrestricted Net Assets (net income)} + \text{Interest, Depreciation, Amortization}}{\text{Maximum Annual Debt Service}}$$

6. Liabilities to Fund Balance

$$\frac{\text{Total Liabilities}}{\text{Unrestricted Fund Balances}}$$

Profitability Ratios

7. Operating Margin (%)

$$\frac{\text{Operating Income (Loss)}}{\text{Total Operating Revenues}}$$

8. Return on Total Assets (%)

$$\frac{\text{EBIT (Earnings before Interest and Taxes)}}{\text{Total Assets}}$$

Courtesy of Resource Group, Ltd., Dallas, Texas.

Liquidity ratios measure short-term sufficiency. As the name implies, they measure the ability of the organization to "be liquid": in other words, to have sufficient cash—or assets that can be converted to cash—on hand.

Current Ratio

The current ratio equals current assets divided by current liabilities. To use the Westside Clinic example in the previous chapter

$$\frac{\text{Current Assets}}{\text{Current Liabilities}} = \frac{\$120,000}{\$60,000} = 2 \text{ to } 1$$

This ratio is considered to be a measure of short-term debt-paying ability. However, it must be carefully interpreted. The standard by which current ratio is measured is 2 to 1, as computed previously.

Quick Ratio

The quick ratio equals cash plus short-term investments plus net receivables divided by current liabilities. In our example,

$$\frac{\text{Cash and Cash Eqivalents} + \text{Net Receivables}}{\text{Current Liabilities}} = \frac{\$65,000}{60,000} = 1.08 \text{ to } 1$$

The standard by which the quick ratio is measured is generally 1 to 1. This computation, at 1.08 to 1, is a little better than the standard.

This ratio is considered to be an even more severe test of short-term debt-paying ability (even more than the current ratio). The quick ratio is also known as the acid-test ratio for obvious reasons.

Days Cash on Hand

The days cash on hand (DCOH) equals unrestricted cash and investments divided by cash operating expenses/365. In our example

$$\frac{\begin{array}{c}\text{Unrestricted Cash and}\\ \text{Cash Equivalents}\end{array}}{\begin{array}{l}\text{Cash Operating Expenses}\\ \div \text{No. of Days in Period}\end{array}} = \frac{\$330,000}{\$11,000} = 30 \text{ days}$$

there is no concrete standard for this computation.

This ratio indicates cash on hand in relation to the amount of daily operating expense. This example indicates the organization has 30 days worth of operating expenses represented in the amount of (unrestricted) cash on hand.

Days Receivables

The days receivables computation is represented as net receivables divided by net credit revenues/365. In our example

$$\frac{\text{Net Receivables}}{\begin{array}{l}\text{Net Credit Revenue/}\\ \text{No. of Days in Period}\end{array}} = \frac{\$720,000}{\$12,000} = 60 \text{ days}$$

This computation represents the number of days in receivables. The older a receivable is, the more difficult it becomes to collect. Therefore, this computation is a measure of worth as well as performance.

There is no hard and fast rule for this computation because much depends on the mix of payers in your organization. This example indicates that the organization has 60 days worth of credit revenue tied up in net receivables. This computation is a common measure of billing and collection performance. There are many "days receivables" regional and national figures to compare with your own organization's computation.

Figure 10–1 shows how the information for the numerator and the denominator of each calculation is obtained. It takes the Westside Clinic balance sheet and the state-ment of revenue and expense that were discussed in the preceding chapter and illus-trates the source of each figure in the four ratios just discussed. The multiple computa-tions for days cash on hand and for days re-ceivables are further broken down into a three-step process. If you study Figure 10–1 and work with the Mini-Case Study, you will own this process.

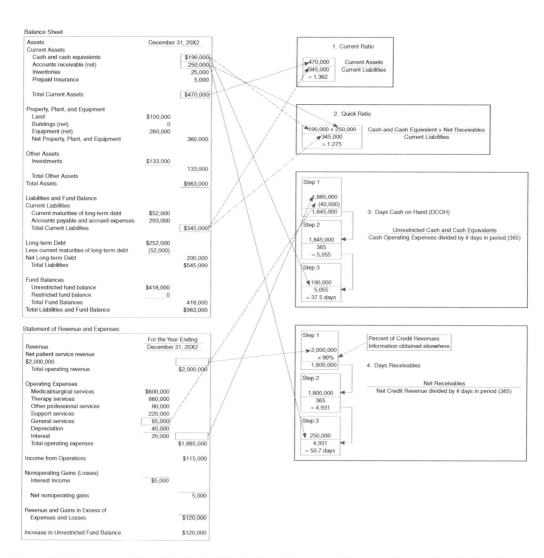

Figure 10–1 Examples of Liquidity Ratio Calculations, Courtesy of Resource Group, Ltd., Dallas, Texas.

SOLVENCY RATIOS

Solvency ratios reflect the ability of the organization to pay the annual interest and principal obligations on its long-term debt. As the name implies, they measure the ability of the organization to "be solvent": in other words, to have sufficient resources to meet its long-term obligations.

Debt Service Coverage Ratio

The debt service coverage ratio (DSCR) is represented as change in unrestricted net assets (net income) plus interest, depreciation, and amortization divided by maximum annual debt service. In our example

$$\frac{\begin{array}{c}\text{Change in Unrestricted}\\ \text{Net Assets (Net Income) +}\\ \text{Interest, Depreciation,}\\ \text{and Amortization}\end{array}}{\begin{array}{c}\text{Maximum Annual Debt}\\ \text{Service}\end{array}} = \frac{\$250,000}{\$100,000} = 2.5$$

This ratio is universally used in credit analysis and figures prominently in the Mini-Case Study.

Each lending institution has its particular criteria for the DSCR. Lending agreements often have a provision that requires the DSCR to be maintained at or above a certain figure.

Liabilities to Fund Balance (or Debt to Net Worth)

The liabilities to fund balance or net worth computation is represented as total liabilities divided by unrestricted net assets (i.e., fund balances or net worth) or total debt divided by tangible net worth. In our example

$$\frac{\text{Total Liabilities}}{\begin{array}{c}\text{Unrestricted Fund}\\ \text{Balances}\end{array}} = \frac{\$2,000,000}{\$2,250,000} = .80$$

This figure is a quick indicator of debt load.

Another indicator that is more severe is long-term debt to net worth (fund balance), which is computed as long-term debt divided by fund balance. This computation is somewhat equivalent to the quick ratio discussed previously here in its restrictiveness to net worth computation.

A mirror image of total liabilities to fund balance is total assets to fund balance, which is computed as total assets divided by fund balance.

Figure 10–2 shows how the information for the numerator and the denominator of each calculation is obtained. This figure again takes the Westside Clinic balance sheet and statement of revenue and expense that were discussed in the preceding chapter and illustrates the source of each figure in the two solvency ratios just discussed, along with each figure in the two profitability ratios still to be discussed. When multiple computations are necessary, they are further broken down into a two-step process.

PROFITABILITY RATIOS

Profitability ratios reflect the ability of the organization to operate with an excess of operating revenue over operating expense. Nonprofit organizations may not call this result a profit, but the measurement ratios are still generally called profitability ratios, whether they are applied to for-profit or nonprofit organizations.

Operating Margin

The operating margin, which is generally expressed as percentage, is represented as operating income (loss) divided by total operating revenues. In our example

$$\frac{\text{Operating Income (Loss)}}{\substack{\text{Total Operating} \\ \text{Revenues}}} = \frac{\$250,000}{\$5,000,000} = 5.0\%$$

This ratio is used for a number of managerial purposes and also sometimes enters

into credit analysis. It is therefore a multipurpose measure. It is so universal that many outside sources are available for comparative purposes. The result of the computation must still be carefully considered because of variables in each period being compared.

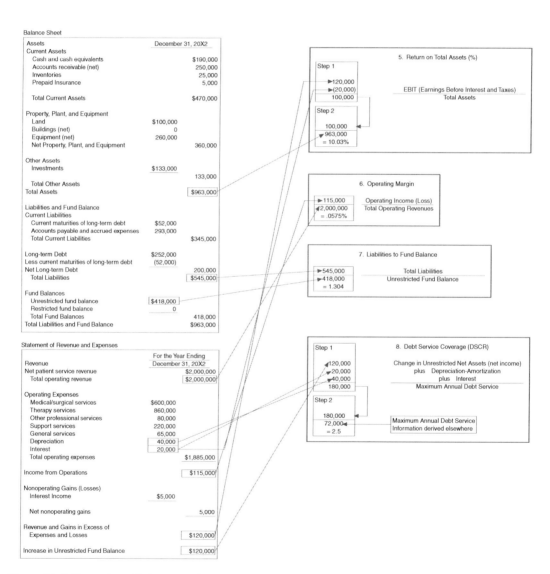

Figure 10–2 Examples of Solvency and Profitability Ratio Calculations. Courtesy of Resource Group, Ltd., Dallas Texas.

Return on Total Assets

The return on total assets is represented as earnings before interest and taxes (EBIT) divided by total assets. In our example

$$\frac{\text{EBIT}}{\text{Total Assets}} = \frac{\$400,000}{\$4,000,000} = 10\%$$

This is a broad measure in common use. Note the acronym *EBIT*, as its use is widespread in credit analysis circles.

This concludes the description of solvency and profitability ratios. Again, if you study Figure 10–2 and work with the Mini-Case Study, you will own this process too.

 INFORMATION CHECKPOINT

What Is Needed?	Reports that use ratios as measures.
Where Is It Found?	Possibly in your supervisor's file; in the administrator's office; in the chief executive officer's office.
How Is It Used?	Use as a measure against outside benchmarks (as discussed in this chapter); also use as internal benchmarks for departments/divisions/units; also use as benchmarks at various points over time.

 KEY TERMS

Current Ratio
Days Cash on Hand (DCOH)
Days Receivables
Debt Service Coverage Ratio (DSCR)
Liabilities to Fund Balance
Liquidity Ratios
Operating Margin
Profitability Ratios
Quick Ratio
Return on Total Assets
Solvency Ratios

 DISCUSSION QUESTIONS

1. Are there ratios in the reports you receive at your workplace?
2. If so, do you use them? How?
3. If not, do you believe ratios should be on the reports? Which reports?
4. Can you think of good outside sources that could be used to obtain ratios for comparative purposes? If the outside information was available, what ratios would you choose to use? Why?

CHAPTER 11

The Time Value of Money

PROGRESS NOTES

After completing this chapter, you should be able to

1. Compute an unadjusted rate of return.
2. Understand how to use a present-value table.
3. Compute an internal rate of return.
4. Understand the payback period theory.

PURPOSE

The purpose of these computations is to evaluate the use of money. The manager has many options as to where resources of the organization should be spent.[1] These calculations provide guides to assist in evaluating the alternatives.

UNADJUSTED RATE OF RETURN

The unadjusted rate of return is a relatively unsophisticated return-on-investment method, and the answer is only an estimate, containing no precision. The computation of the unadjusted rate of return is as follows:

$$\frac{\text{average annual net income}}{\text{original investment amount}} = \text{rate of return}$$

OR

$$\frac{\text{average annual net income}}{\text{average investment amount}} = \text{rate of return}$$

The original investment amount is a matter of record. The average investment amount is arrived at by taking the total unrecovered asset cost at the beginning of estimated useful life plus the unrecovered asset cost at the end of estimated useful life and dividing by two. This method has the advantage of accommodating whatever depreciation method has been chosen by the organization. This method is sometimes called the accountant's method because information necessary for the computation is obtained from the financial statements.

PRESENT-VALUE ANALYSIS

The concept of present-value analysis is based on the time value of money. Inherent in this concept is the fact that the value of a dollar today is more than the value of a dollar in the future: thus the "present value" terminology. Furthermore, the further in the future the receipt of your dollar occurs, the less it is worth. Think of a dollar bill dwindling in size more and more as its receipt stretches further and further into the future. This is the concept of present-value analysis.

We learned about compound interest in math class. We learned that

$500   invested at the beginning of year 1
 .05   earns interest (assumed) at a rate of
____   5% for one year,
$525   and we have a compound amount at
       the end of year 1 amounting to $525,
 .05   which earns interest (assumed) at the
____   rate of 5% for another year,
$551   and we have a compound amount at
       the end of year 2 amounting to $551
       (rounded), and so on.

Using this concept, it is possible to restate the present values of $1 to be paid out or received at the end of each of these years. It is possible to use equations, but that is not necessary because we have present value tables (also called "look-up tables," because one can "look-up" the answer). A present value table is included at the end of this chapter in Appendix 11–A. All of the figures on the present value table represent the value of a dollar. The interest rate available on this version of the table is on the horizontal columns and ranges from 1 percent to 50 percent. The number of years in the period is on the vertical; in this version of the table, the number of years ranges from 1 to 30. To look up a present value, find the column for the proper interest. Then find the line for the proper number of years. Then trace down the interest column and across the number-of-years line item. The point where the two lines meet is the number (or factor) that represents the value of $1 according to your assumptions. For example, find the year 10 by reading down the left-hand col-

umn labeled "Year." Then read across that line until you find the column labeled "10%." The point where the two lines meet is found to be 0.3855. The present value of $1 under these assumptions (10 year/10%) is about 38.5 cents.

Besides using the look-up table, you can also compute this factor on a business calculator. The computation instructions are contained in Appendix B at the back of this book.

Besides using either the look-up table or the business calculator, you can use a function on your computer spreadsheet to produce the factor. The important point is this: no matter which method you use, you should get the same answer.

Now that you have the present value of $1, by whichever method, it is simple to find the present value of any other number. You merely multiply the other number by the factor you found on the table—or in the calculator or the computer. Say, for example, you want to find the present value of $8,000 under the assumption used above (10 years/10%). You simply multiply $8,000 by the factor of 0.3855 you found in the table. The present value of $8,000 is $3,084 (or $8,000 times 0.3855). A compound interest table is also included at the end of this chapter in Appendix 11–B so that you have the tools for computation at your disposal.

INTERNAL RATE OF RETURN

The internal rate of return (IRR) is another return on investment method. It uses a discounted cash flow technique. The internal rate of return is the rate of interest that discounts future net inflows (from the proposed investment) down to the amount invested. The return for a particular investment can therefore be known. The IRR recognizes the elements contained in the previous two methods discussed, but it goes further. It also recognizes the time pattern in which the earnings occur. This means more precision in the computation because IRR calculates from period to period, whereas the other two methods rely on an average investment.

The IRR computation is not very complicated. The computation requires two assumptions and three steps to compute. Assumption 1: find the initial cost of the investment. Assumption 2: find the estimated annual net cash inflow the investment will generate. Assumption 3: find the useful life of the asset (generally expressed in number of years, known as periods for this computation). Step 1: Divide the initial cost of the investment (assumption 1) by the estimated annual net cash inflow it will generate (assumption 2). The answer is a ratio. Step 2: Now use the look-up table. Find the number of periods (assumption 3). Step 3: Look across the line for the number of periods and find the column that approximates the ratio computed in Step 1. That column contains the interest rate representing the rate of return.

How is IRR used? It can take the rate of return obtained and restate it. The restated figure represents the maximum rate of interest that can be paid for capital over the entire span of the investment without incurring a loss. (You can think of that restated figure as a kind of breakeven point for investment purposes.) The fact that a rate of return can be computed is the benefit of using an IRR method.

PAYBACK PERIOD

The payback period is the length of time required for the cash coming in from an investment to equal the amount of cash originally spent when the investment was acquired. In other words, if we invested $1,000, under a particular set of assumptions, how long would it take to get our $1,000 back? The payback period concept is used extensively in evaluating whether to invest in plant and/or equipment. In that case, the question can be restated as follows: If we invested $1,200,000 in a magnetic resonance imaging machine, under a particular set of assumptions, how long would it take to get the hospital's $1,200,000 back?

The assumptions are key to the computation of the payback period. In the case of equipment, volume of usage is a critical assumption and is sometimes very difficult to predict. Therefore, it is prudent to run more than one payback period computation based on different circumstances. Generally a "best case" and a "worst case" run are made.

The computation itself is simple, although it has multiple steps. The trick is to break it into segments.

For example, Doctor Green is considering the purchase of a machine for his office laboratory. It will cost $300,000. He wants to find the payback period for this piece of equipment. To begin Dr. Green needs to make the following assumptions: Assumption 1: Purchase price of the equipment. Assumption 2: Useful life of the equipment. Assumption 3: Revenue the machine will generate per year. Assumption 4: Direct operating costs associated with earning the revenue. Assumption 5: Depreciation expense per year (computed as purchase price per assumption 1 divided by useful life per assumption 2).

Dr. Green's five assumptions are as follows:

1. Purchase price of equipment = $300,000
2. Useful life of the equipment = 10 years

3. Revenue the machine will generate per year = $10,000 after taxes
4. Direct operating costs associated with earning the revenue = $150,000
5. Depreciation expense per year = $30,000

Now that the assumptions are in place, the payback period computation can be made. It is in three steps, as follows:

Step 1: Find the machine's expected net income after taxes:

Revenue (assumption #3)	$200,000
Less	
Direct operating costs	
(assumption #4) $150,000	
Depreciation	
(assumption #5) 30,000	
	180,000
Net income before taxes	$20,000
Less income taxes of 50%	10,000
Net income after taxes	$10,000

Step 2: Find the net annual cash inflow after taxes the machine is expected to generate (in other words, convert the net income to a cash basis):

Net income after taxes	$10,000
Add back depreciation	
(a noncash expenditure)	30,000
Annual net cash inflow after taxes	$40,000

Step 3: Compute the payback period:

$$\frac{\text{investment } \$300,000 \text{ machine cost*}}{\text{net annual cash flow after taxes } \$40,000**} = \begin{array}{l} 7.5 \\ \text{year} \\ \text{pay-} \\ \text{back} \\ \text{period} \end{array}$$

*assumption 1 above
**per step 2 above

The machine will pay back its investment under these assumptions in 7.5 years.

Payback period computations are very common when equipment purchases are being evaluated. The evaluation process itself is the final subject we consider in this chapter.

EVALUATIONS

Evaluating the use of resources in health care organizations is an important task. There are never enough resources to go around, and it is important to use an objective process to evaluate which investments will be made by the organization. A uniform use of a chosen method of evaluating return on investment and/or payback period makes the evaluation process more manageable.

It is important to choose a method that is understood by the managers who will be using it. It is equally important to choose a method that can be readily calculated. If a multiple-page worksheet has to be constructed to set up the assumptions for a modestly priced piece of equipment, the evaluation method is probably too complex. This comment actually touches on the cost-benefit of performing the evaluation.

Sometimes a computer program is chosen that performs a uniform computation of investment returns and payback periods. Such a program is a suitable choice if the managers who use it understand the printouts it produces. Understanding both input and output is key for the managers. In summary, evaluations should be objective, the process should not be too cumbersome, and the responsible managers should understand how the computation was achieved.

INFORMATION CHECKPOINT

What Is Needed?	Information sufficient to perform these calculations.
Where Is It Found?	In the files of your supervisor; also in the office of the financial analyst; probably also in the strategic planning office.
How Is It Used?	To measure the time value of money

 KEY TERMS

Internal Rate of Return
Payback Period
Present Value Analysis
Time Value of Money
Unadjusted Rate of Return

 DISCUSSION QUESTIONS

1. Can you compute an unadjusted rate of return now? Would you use it? Why?
2. Are you able to use the present-value look-up table now? Would you prefer a computer to compute it?
3. Have you seen the payback period concept used in your workplace? If not, do you think it ought to be used? What are your reasons?
4. Have you had a chance to participate in an evaluation of an equipment purchase at your workplace? If so, would you have done it differently if you had supervised the evaluation? Why?

Present Value Table

(The Present Value of $1.00)

Year	1%	2%	3%	4%	5%	6%	7%	8%	9%	10%
1	0.9901	0.9804	0.9709	0.9615	0.9524	0.9434	0.9346	0.9259	0.9174	0.9091
2	0.9803	0.9612	0.9426	0.9246	0.9070	0.8900	0.8734	0.8573	0.8417	0.8264
3	0.9706	0.9423	0.9151	0.8890	0.8638	0.8396	0.8163	0.7938	0.7722	0.7513
4	0.9610	0.9238	0.8885	0.8548	0.8227	0.7921	0.7629	0.7350	0.7084	0.6830
5	0.9515	0.9057	0.8626	0.8219	0.7835	0.7473	0.7130	0.6806	0.6499	0.6209
6	0.9420	0.8880	0.8375	0.7903	0.7462	0.7050	0.6663	0.6302	0.5963	0.5645
7	0.9327	0.8706	0.8131	0.7599	0.7107	0.6651	0.6227	0.5835	0.5470	0.5132
8	0.9235	0.8535	0.7894	0.7307	0.6768	0.6274	0.5820	0.5403	0.5019	0.4665
9	0.9143	0.8368	0.7664	0.7026	0.6446	0.5919	0.5439	0.5002	0.4604	0.4241
10	0.9053	0.8203	0.7441	0.6756	0.6139	0.5584	0.5083	0.4632	0.4224	0.3855
11	0.8963	0.8043	0.7224	0.6496	0.5847	0.5268	0.4751	0.4289	0.3875	0.3505
12	0.8874	0.7885	0.7014	0.6246	0.5568'	0.4970	0.4440	0.3971	0.3555	0.3186
13	0.8787	0.7730	0.6810	0.6006	0.5303	0.4688	0.4150	0.3677	0.3262	0.2987
14	0.8700	0.7579	0.6611	0.5775	0.5051	0.4423	0.3878	0.3405	0.2992	0.2633
15	0.8613	0.7430	0.6419	0.5553	0.4810	0.4173	0.3624	0.3152	0.2745	0.2394
16	0.8528	0.7284	0.6232	0.5339	0.4581	0.3936	0.3387	0.2919	0.2519	0.2176
17	0.8444	0.7142	0.6050	0.5134	0.4363	0.3714	0.3166	0.2703	0.2311	0.1978
18	0.8360	0.7002	0.5874	0.4936	0.4155	0.3503	0.2959	0.2502	0.2120	0.1799
19	0.8277	0.6864	0.5703	0.4746	0.3957	0.3305	0.2765	0.2317.	0.1945	0.1635
20	0.8195	0.6730	0.5537	0.4564	0.3769	0.3118	0.2584	0.2145	0.1784	0.1486
21	0.8114	0.6598	0.5375	0.4388	0.3589	0.2942	0.2415	0.1987	0.1637	0.1351
22	0.8034	0.6468	0.5219	0.4220	0.3418	0.2775	0.2257	0.1839	0.1502	0.1228
23	0.7954	0.6342	0.5067	0.4057	0.3256	0.2618	0.2109	0.1703	0.1378	0.1117
24	0.7876	0.6217	0.4919	0.3901	0.3101	0.2470	0.1971	0.1577	0.1264	0.1015
25	0.7798	0.6095	0.4776	0.3751	0.2953	0.2330	0.1842	0.1460	0.1160	0.0923
26	0.7720	0.5976	0.4637	0.3607	0.2812	0.2198	0.1722	0.1352	0.1064	0.0839
27	0.7644	0.5859	0.4502	0.3468	0.2678	0.2074	0.1609	0.1252	0.0976	0.0763
28	0.7568	0.5744	0.4371	0.3335	0.2552	0.1956	0.1504	0.1159	0.0895	0.0693
29	0.7493	0.5631	0.4243	0.3207	0.2429	0.1846	0.1406	0.1073	0.0822	0.0630
30	0.7419	0.5521	0.4120	0.3083	0.2314	0.1741	0.1314	0.0994	0.0754	0.0573

Year	11%	12%	13%	14%	15%	16%	17%	18%	19%	20%
1	0.9009	0.8929	0.8850	0.8772	0.8696	0.8621	0.8547	0.8475	0.8403	0.8333
2	0.8116	0.7972	0.7831	0.7695	0.7561	0.7432	0.7305	0.7182	0.7062	0.6944
3	0.7312	0.7118	0.6913	0.6750	0.6575	0.6407	0.6244	0.6086	0.5934	0.5787
4	0.6587	0.6355	0.6133	0.5921	0.5718	0.5523	0.5337	0.5158	0.4987	0.4823
5	0.5935	0.5674	0.5428	0.5194	0.4972	0.4761	0.4561	0.4371	0.4190	0.4019
6	0.5346	0.5066	0.4803	0.4556	0.4323	0.4104	0.3898	0.3704	0.3521	0.3349
7	0.4817	0.4523	0.4251	0.3996	0.3759	0.3538	0.3332	0.3139	0.2959	0.2791
8	0.4339	0.4039	0.3762	0.3506	0.3269	0.3050	0.2848	0.2660	0.2487	0.2326
9	0.3909	0.3606	0.3329	0.3075	0.2843	0.2630	0.2434	0.2255	0.2090	0.1938
10	0.3522	0.3220	0.2946	0.2697	0.2472	0.2267	0.2080	0.1911	0.1756	0.1615
11	0.3173	0.2875	0.2607	0.2366	0.2149	0.1954	0.1778	0.1619	0.1476	0.1346
12	0.2858	0.2567	0.2307	0.2076	0.1869	0.1685	0.1520	0.1372	0.1240	0.1122
13	0.2575	0.2292	0.2042	0.1821	0.1625	0.1452	0.1299	0.1163	0.1042	0.0935
14	0.2320	0.2046	0.1807	0.1597	0.1413	0.1252	0.1110	0.0985	0.0876	0.0779
15	0.2090	0.1827	0.1599	0.1401	0.1229	0.1079	0.0949	0.0835	0.0736	0.0649
16	0.1883	0.1631	0.1415	0.1229	0.1069	0.0930	0.0811	0.0708	0.0618	0.0541
17	0.1696	0.1456	0.1252	0.1078	0.0929	0.0802	0.0693	0.0600	0.0520	0.0451
18	0.1528	0.1300	0.1108	0.0946	0.0808	0.0691	0.0592	0.0508	0.0437	0.0376
19	0.1377	0.1161	0.0981	0.0829	0.0703	0.0596	0.0506	0.0431	0.0367	0.0313
20	0.1240	0.1037	0.0868	0.0728	0.0611	0.0514	0.0433	0.0365	0.0308	0.0261
21	0.1117	0.0926	0.0768	0.0638	0.0531	0.0443	0.0370	0.0309	0.0259	0.0217
22	0.1007	0.0826	0.0680	0.0560	0.0462	0.0382	0.0316	0.0262	0.0218	0.0181
23	0.0907	0.0738	0.0601	0.0491	0.0402	0.0329	0.0270	0.0222	0.0183	0.0151
24	0.0817	0.0659	0.0532	0.0431	0.0349	0.0284	0.0231	0.0188	0.0154	0.0126
25	0.0736	0.0588	0.0471	0.0378	0.0304	0.0245	0.0197	0.0160	0.0129	0.0105
26	0.0663	0.0525	0.0417	0.0331	0.0264	0.0211	0.0169	0.0135	0.0109	0.0087
27	0.0597	0.0469	0.0369	0.0291	0.0230	0.0182	0.0144	0.0115	0.0091	0.0073
28	0.0538	0.0419	0.0326	0.0255	0.0200	0.0157	0.0123	0.0097	0.0077	0.0061
29	0.0485	0.0374	0.0289	0.0224	0.0174	0.0135	0.0105	0.0082	0.0064	0.0051
30	0.0437	0.0334	0.0256	0.0196	0.0151	0.0116	0.0090	0.0070	0.0054	0.0042

Compound Interest Table
Compound Interest of $1.00
(The Future Amount of $1.00)

Year	1%	2%	3%	4%	5%	6%	7%	8%	9%	10%
1	1.010	1.020	1.030	1.040	1.050	1.060	1.070	1.080	1.090	1.100
2	1.020	1.040	1.061	1.082	1.102	1.124	1.145	1.166	1.188	1.210
3	1.030	1.061	1.093	1.125	1.156	1.191	1.225	1.260	1.295	1.331
4	1.041	1.082	1.126	1.170	1.216	1.262	1.311	1.360	1.412	1.464
5	1.051	1.104	1.159	1.217	1.276	1.338	1.403	1.469	1.539	1.611
6	1.062	1.120	1.194	1.265	1.340	1.419	1.501	1.587	1.677	1.772
7	1.072	1.149	1.230	1.316	1.407	1.504	1.606	1.714	1.828	1.949
8	1.083	1.172	1.267	1.369	1.477	1.594	1.718	1.851	1.993	2.144
9	1.094	1.195	1.305	1.423	1.551	1.689	1.838	1.999	2.172	2.358
10	1.105	1.219	1.344	1.480	1.629	1.791	1.967	2.159	2.367	2.594
11	1.116	1.243	1.384	1.539	1.710	1.898	2.105	2.332	2.580	2.853
12	1.127	1.268	1.426	1.601	1.796	2.012	2.252	2.518	2.813	3.138
13	1.138	1.294	1.469	1.665	1.886	2.133	2.410	2.720	3.066	3.452
14	1.149	1.319	1.513	1.732	1.980	2.261	2.579	2.937	3.342	3.797
15	1.161	1.346	1.558	1.801	2.079	2.397	2.759	3.172	3.642	4.177
16	1.173	1.373	1.605	1.873	2.183	2.540	2.952	3.426	3.970	4.595
17	1.184	1.400	1.653	1.948	2.292	2.693	3.159	3.700	4.328	5.054
18	1.196	1.428	1.702	2.026	2.407	2.854	3.380	3.996	4.717	5.560
19	1.208	1.457	1.754	2.107	2.527	3.026	3.617	4.316	5.142	6.116
20	1.220	1.486	1.806	2.191	2.653	3.207	3.870	4.661	5.604	6.728
25	1.282	1.641	2.094	2.666	3.386	4.292	5.427	6.848	8.632	10.835
30	1.348	1.811	2.427	3.243	4.322	5.743	7.612	10.063	13.268	17.449

Year	12%	14%	16%	18%	20%	24%	28%	32%	40%	50%
1	1.120	1.140	1.160	1.180	1.200	1.240	1.280	1.320	1.400	1.500
2	1.254	1.300	1.346	1.392	1.440	1.538	1.638	1.742	1.960	2.250
3	1.405	1.482	1.561	1.643	1.728	1.907	2.067	2.300	2.744	3.375
4	1.574	1.689	1.811	1.939	2.074	2.364	2.684	3.036	3.842	5.062
5	1.762	1.925	2.100	2.288	2.488	2.932	3.436	4.007	5.378	7.594
6	1.974	2.195	2.436	2.700	2.986	3.635	4.398	5.290	7.530	11.391
7	2.211	2.502	2.826	3.185	3.583	4.508	5.629	6.983	10.541	17.086
8	2.476	2.853	3.278	3.759	4.300	5.590	7.206	9.217	14.758	25.629
9	2.773	3.252	3.803	4.435	5.160	6.931	9.223	12.166	20.661	38.443
10	3.106	3.707	4.411	5.234	6.192	8.594	11.806	16.060	28.925	57.665
11	3.479	4.226	5.117	6.176	7.430	10.657	15.112	21.199	40.496	86.498
12	3.896	4.818	5.936	7.288	8.916	13.215	19.343	27.983	56.694	129.746
13	4.363	5.492	6.886	8.599	10.699	16.386	24.759	36.937	79.372	194.619
14	4.887	6.261	7.988	10.147	12.839	20.319	31.691	48.757	111.120	291.929
15	5.474	7.138	9.266	11.074	15.407	25.196	40.565	64.350	155.568	437.894
16	6.130	8.137	10.748	14.129	18.488	31.243	51.923	84.954	217.795	656.840
17	6.866	9.276	12.468	16.672	22.186	38.741	66.461	112.140	304.914	985.260
18	7.690	10.575	14.463	19.673	26.623	48.039	85.071	148.020	426.879	1477.900
19	8.613	12.056	16.777	23.214	31.948	59.568	108.890	195.390	597.630	2216.800
20	9.646	13.743	19.461	27.393	38.338	73.864	139.380	257.920	836.683	3325.300
25	17.000	26.462	40.874	62.669	95.396	216.542	478.900	1033.600	4499.880	25251.000
30	29.960	50.950	85.850	143.371	237.376	634.820	1645.500	4142.100	24201.432	191750.000

Present Value of an Annuity of $1.00

Periods	2%	4%	6%	8%	10%	12%	14%	16%	18%	20%	Periods
1	.980	.962	.943	.926	.909	.893	.877	.862	.848	.833	1
2	1.942	1.886	1.833	1.783	1.736	1.690	1.647	1.605	1.566	1.528	2
3	2.884	2.775	2.673	2.577	2.487	2.402	2.322	2.246	2.174	2.107	3
4	3.808	3.630	3.465	3.312	3.170	3.037	2.914	2.798	2.690	2.589	4
5	4.713	4.452	4.212	3.993	3.791	3.605	3.433	3.274	3.127	2.991	5
6	5.601	5.242	4.917	4.623	4.355	4.111	3.889	3.685	3.498	3.326	6
7	6.472	6.002	5.582	5.206	4.868	4.564	4.288	4.039	3.812	3.605	7
8	7.325	6.733	6.210	5.747	5.335	4.968	4.639	4.344	4.078	3.837	8
9	8.162	7.435	6.802	6.247	5.759	5.328	4.946	4.607	4.303	4.031	9
10	8.983	8.111	7.360	6.710	6.145	5.650	5.216	4.833	4.494	4.193	10
15	12.849	11.118	9.712	8.560	7.606	6.811	6.142	5.576	5.092	4.676	15
20	16.351	13.590	11.470	9.818	8.514	7.469	6.623	5.929	5.353	4.870	20
25	19.523	15.622	12.783	10.675	9.077	7.843	6.873	6.097	5.467	4.948	25

PART V

Plan, Monitor, and Control Financial Operations

Comparative Data, Forecasts, and Benchmarking

COMPARATIVE DATA

Purpose

Comparative analysis is important to managers because it creates a common ground to make judgments for planning, control, and decision-making purposes.

Common Sizing

The process of common sizing puts information on the same relative basis. Generally, common sizing involves converting dollar amounts to percentages. If, for example, total revenue of $200,000 equals 100 percent, then radiology revenue of $20,000 will equal 10 percent of that total. Converting dollars to percentages allows comparative analysis. In other words, comparing the percentages allows a common basis of comparison. Common sizing is sometimes called *vertical analysis* (because the computation of the percentages is vertical).

Although such comparisons on the basis of percentages can and should be performed on your own organization's data, comparisons can also be made between or among various organizations. For example, Table 12–1 shows how common sizing allows a comparison of liabilities for three different hospitals. In each case, the total liabilities equal 100 percent. Then the current liabilities of hospital 1, for example, are divided by total liabilities to find the proportionate percentage attributable to that line item (100,000 divided by 500,000 equals 20 percent; 400,000 divided by 500,000 equals 80 percent). When all the percentages have been computed, add them to make sure they add to 100 percent. If you use a computer, computation of these percentages is available as a spreadsheet function.

Another example of comparative analysis is contained in Table 12–2. In this case, gen-

Table 12–1 Common Sizing Liability Information

| | Same Year for All Three Hospitals | | | | | |
	Hospital 1		Hospital 2		Hospital 3	
Current liabilities	$100,000	20%	$500,000	25%	$400,000	80%
Long-term debt	400,000	80%	1,500,000	75%	100,000	20%
Total liabilities	$500,000	100%	$2,000,000	100%	$500,000	100%

eral services expenses for three hospitals are compared. Once again, the total expense for each hospital becomes 100 percent, and the relative percentage for each of the four line items is computed ($320,000 divided by $800,000 equals 40 percent and so on). The advantage of comparative analysis is illustrated by the "laundry" line item, where the dollar amounts are $80,000, $300,000, and $90,000 respectively. Yet each of these amounts is 10 percent of the total expense for the particular hospital.

Trend Analysis

The process of trend analysis compares figures over several time periods. Once again, dollar amounts are converted to percentages to obtain a relative basis for purposes of comparison, but now the comparison is across time. If, for example, radiology revenue was $20,000 this period but was only $15,000 for the previous period, the difference between the two is $5,000. The difference of $5,000 equates to a 33⅓ percent difference because trend analysis is computed on the earlier of the two years: that is, the base year (thus, 5,000 divided by 15,000 equals 33⅓ percent). Trend analysis is sometimes called *horizontal analysis* (because the computation of the percentage of difference is horizontal).

An example of horizontal analysis is contained in Table 12–3. In this case, the liabilities of hospital 1 for year 1 are compared with the liabilities of hospital 1's year 2. Current liabilities, for example, were $100,000 in year 1 and are $150,000 in year 2, a difference of $50,000. To arrive at a percentage of difference for comparative purposes, the $50,000 difference is divided by the year 1 base figure of $100,000 to compute the relative differential (thus, 50,000 divided by 100,000 is 50 percent).

Table 12–2 Common Sizing Expense Information

| | Same Year for All Three Hospitals | | | | | |
	Hospital 1		Hospital 2		Hospital 3	
General services expense						
Dietary	$320,000	40%	$1,260,000	42%	$450,000	50%
Maintenance	280,000	35%	990,000	33%	135,000	15%
Laundry	80,000	10%	300,000	10%	90,000	10%
Housekeeping	120,000	15%	450,000	15%	225,000	25%
Total GS expense	$800,000	100%	$3,000,000	100%	$900,000	100%

Table 12–3 Trend Analysis for Liabilities

	Hospital 1					
	Year 1		Year 2		Difference	
Current liabilities	$100,000	20%	$150,000	25%	$50,000	50%
Long-term debt	400,000	80%	450,000	75%	50,000	12.5%
Total liabilities	$500,000	100%	$600,000	100%	$100,000	–

Another example of comparative analysis is contained in Table 12–4. In this case, general services expenses for two years in hospital 1 are compared. The difference between year 1 and year 2 for each line item is computed in dollars; then the dollar difference figure is divided by the year 1 base figure to obtain a percentage difference for purposes of comparison. Thus, housekeeping expense in year 1 was $120,000, and in year 2, was $180,000, resulting in a difference of $60,000. The difference amounts to 50 percent ($60,000 difference divided by $120,000 year 1 equals 50 percent). In Table 12–4 two of the four line items have negative differences: that is, year 2 was less than year 1, resulting in a negative figure. Also, the dollar figure difference is $100,000 when added down (subtract the negative figures from the positive figures; thus, $85,000 plus $60,000 minus $10,000 minus $35,000 equals $100,000). The dollar figure difference is also $100,000 when added across ($900,000 minus $800,000 equals $100,000).

Analyzing Operating Data

Comparative analysis is an important tool for managers, and it is worth investing the time to become familiar with both horizontal and vertical analysis. Managers will generally analyze their own organization's data most of the time (rather than performing comparisons against other organizations). With that fact in mind, we examine operating room operating data (no pun intended) that incorporate both common sizing and trend analysis.

Table 12–5 sets out 32 expense items. The expense amount in dollars for each line item is set out for the current year in the left column (beginning with $60,517). The

Table 12–4 Trend Analysis for Expenses

	Hospital 1					
	Year 1		Year 2		Difference	
General services expense						
Dietary	$320,000	40%	$405,000	45%	$85,000	26.5%
Maintenance	280,000	35%	270,000	30%	(10,000)	(3.5)%
Laundry	80,000	10%	45,000	5%	(35,000)	(43.5)%
Housekeeping	120,000	15%	180,000	20%	60,000	50.0%
Total GS expense	$800,000	100%	$900,000	100%	$100,000	–

Table 12–5 Vertical and Horizontal Analysis for the Operating Room

	Comparative Expenses					
Account	12-Month Current Year	%	12-Month Prior Year	%	Annual Increase (Decrease)	% of Change
Social Security	60,517	4.97	68,177	5.70	(7,660)	−12.66
Pension	20,675	1.70	23,473	1.96	(2,798)	−13.53
Health Insurance	8,422	0.69	18,507	1.55	(10,085)	−119.75
Child Care	4,564	0.37	4,334	0.36	230	5.04
Patient Accounting	155,356	12.76	123,254	10.30	32,102	20.66
Admitting	110,254	9.05	101,040	8.45	9,214	8.36
Medical Records	91,718	7.53	94,304	7.88	(2,586)	−2.82
Dietary	27,526	2.26	35,646	2.98	(8,120)	−29.50
Medical Waste	2,377	0.20	3,187	0.27	(810)	−34.08
Sterile Procedures	78,720	6.46	70,725	5.91	7,995	10.16
Laundry	40,693	3.34	40,463	3.38	230	0.57
Depreciation—Equipment	87,378	7.18	61,144	5.11	26,234	30.02
Depreciation—Building	41,377	3.40	45,450	3.80	(4,073)	−9.84
Amortization—Interest	(5,819)	−0.48	1,767	0.15	(7,586)	130.37
Insurance	4,216	0.35	7,836	0.65	(3,620)	−85.86
Administration	57,966	4.76	56,309	4.71	1,657	2.86
Medical Staff	1,722	0.14	5,130	0.43	(3,408)	−197.91
Community Relations	49,813	4.09	40,618	3.39	9,195	18.46
Materials Management	64,573	5.30	72,305	6.04	(7,732)	−11.97
Human Resources	31,066	2.55	13,276	1.11	17,790	57.27
Nursing Administration	82,471	6.77	92,666	7.75	(10,195)	−12.36
Data Processing	17,815	1.46	16,119	1.35	1,696	9.52
Fiscal	17,700	1.45	16,748	1.40	952	5.38
Telephone	2,839	0.23	2,569	0.21	270	9.51
Utilities	26,406	2.17	38,689	3.23	(12,283)	−46.52
Plant	77,597	6.37	84,128	7.03	(6,531)	−8.42
Environmental Services	32,874	2.70	37,354	3.12	(4,480)	−13.63
Safety	2,016	0.17	2,179	0.18	(163)	−8.09
Quality Management	10,016	0.82	8,146	0.68	1,870	18.67
Medical Staff	9,444	0.78	9,391	0.78	53	0.56
Continuous Quality Improvement	4,895	0.40	0	0.00	4,895	100.00
EE Health	569	0.05	1,513	0.13	(944)	−165.91
Total Allocated	1,217,756	100.00	1,196,447	100.00	21,309	1.75
All Other Expenses	1,211,608	—	—	—	—	—
Total Expense	2,429,364	—	—	—	—	—

expense amount in dollars for each line item is set out for the prior year in the third column of the analysis (beginning with $68,177). The difference in dollars, labeled "Annual Increase (Decrease)," appears in the sixth column of the analysis (beginning with ($7,660)). Vertical analysis has been performed for the current year, and the percentage results appear in the second column (beginning with 4.97%). Vertical analysis has also been performed for the prior year, and those percentage results appear in the fourth column (beginning with 5.70%). Horizontal analysis has been performed on each line item, and those percentage items appear in the far right column (beginning with –12.66%). This table is a good example of the type of operating data reports that managers receive for planning and control purposes.

FORECASTS

Manager's Use of Forecasts

Forecasted data are information used for purposes of planning for the future. Forecasts can be short range (next year), intermediate range (five years from today), or long range (the next decade and beyond). Forecasting, to some degree or another, is often required when producing budgets. (Budgets are the subject of the next chapter.) It is pretty simple today to create "what if" scenarios on the computer. But the important thing for managers to remember is that assumptions directly affect the results of forecasts.

How Assumptions Affect Forecasted Results

Assumptions Determined by Trend Analysis

One of the basic purposes of performing trend analysis is to compare data between or among years and to see the trends. If such trends are found, then it makes sense to take them into account in your forecast. A word of warning, however: the manager must determine whether the data used for comparison in the trend analysis are comparable data.

Assumptions Determined by Payer Changes

Trend analysis is retrospective: that is, it is using historical data from a past period.

Forecasting is prospective: that is, it is projecting into the future. If changes, say, in regulatory requirements for payment are made this year, then that fact has to be taken into account. Mini-Case Study 2 in Chapter 20 addresses this situation.

Assumptions Determined by Utilization Changes

In health care, significant changes in utilization patterns can be occurring that need to be taken into account in the manager's forecast assumptions. The inexorable shift to shorter lengths of stay for hospital inpatients over the last decade is an example of a basic shift in utilization patterns. Mini-Case Study 2 also addresses this situation.

Staffing Forecasts

Staffing forecasts are a very common type of forecast required of managers. There are three particular pitfalls to be recognized in preparing staffing forecasts: noncontrollable expenses, capacity issues, and labor market issues.

Controllable Versus Noncontrollable Expenses

The concept of responsibility centers and controllable versus noncontrollable expenses has been discussed earlier in this book. Essentially, controllable costs are subject to a manager's own decision making, whereas noncontrollable costs are outside that manager's power. It is extremely difficult to make staffing forecasts with any degree of accuracy if noncontrollable expenses are included in the manager's forecast. The organization's structure must be recognized and taken into account when setting up assumptions for staffing forecasts. Shared services across lines of authority are workable in theory but often do not work in actuality. Figure 12–1 gives an example of the essential

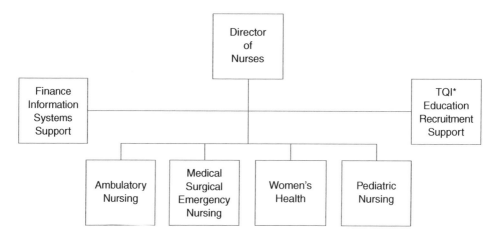

Figure 12–1 Primary Nursing staff Classification by Line of Authority. Courtesy of Resource Group, Ltd., Dallas, Texas.

"business units" under the supervision of a director of nurses. Note the responsibility centers and the support centers on this organization chart.

Capacity Issues in Staffing Forecasts

Capacity is a tricky assumption to make in staffing forecasts. In some programs, particularly those in a startup phase, overcapacity (too much staff available for the amount of work required) is a problem. In some other organizations, undercapacity (a chronic lack of adequate staff) is the problem. Forecasting assumptions, in the best of all worlds, take these difficulties into account. Mini-Case Study 3 in Chapter 21 deals with this problem of staffing in the context of a Women, Infants, and Children (WIC) program.[1]

Labor Market Issues in Staffing Forecasts

The mention of a chronic lack of adequate staff in the preceding paragraph leads us to the problem of the labor market. Certain parts of the country have a continual shortage of certain qualified professional health care staff. Yet other parts of the country can have an overabundance during that same period. The status of the local labor market has a direct impact on staffing forecasts. The impact is in dollars: when there are plenty of staff available, the hourly rate to attract staff goes down, but when there is a shortage of available qualified staff, the hourly rate has to go up. As strange as it may seem, this elemental economic fact is sometimes not taken into account in forecasting assumptions. In summary, the ultimate accuracy of a forecast rests on the strength of its assumptions.

IMPORTANCE OF A VARIETY OF PERFORMANCE MEASURES

If operations are to be managed most effectively, a variety of performance measures must be in place for the organization. Generally a broad variety of such measures are available, and different organizations tend to lean toward using one type over another. One health care organization, for example, may rely heavily on one type of measure, whereas another organization may rely on a very different measurement profile. Generally speaking, a wider variety of performance measures are evident in organizations that have adopted total quality improvement (TQI).

ADJUSTED PERFORMANCE MEASURES OVER TIME

We have previously discussed how measures over time are very effective. The example given in Figure 12–2 combines measures over time with a two-part case mix adjustment. (*Case mix adjustment* refers to adjusting for the acuity level of the patient. It may also refer to the level of resources required to provide care for the patient with the acuity level.) In this case, the desired measure is cost per discharge. The vertical axis is cost in dollars. The horizontal axis is time, a five-year span in this case. Two lines are plotted:

the first is unadjusted for case mix, and the second is case mix adjusted. The unadjusted line rises over the five-year period. However, when the case mix adjustment is taken into account, the plotted line flattens out over time.

BENCHMARKING

Benchmarking is the continuous process of measuring products, services, and activities against the best levels of performance. These best levels may be found inside the organization or outside it. Benchmarks are used to measure performance gaps.

There are three types of benchmarks:

1. A financial variable reported in an accounting system
2. A financial variable not reported in an accounting system
3. A nonfinancial variable

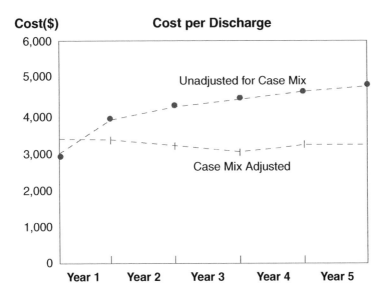

Figure 12–2 Adjusted Performance Measures Over Time.

How to Benchmark

The benchmarking method is predicated on the assumption that an exemplary process, similar to the process being examined, can be identified and examined to establish criteria for excellence. Benchmarking can be accomplished in one of several ways, including (1) studying the methods and end results of your prime competitors, (2) examining the analogous process of noncompetitors with a world-class reputation, or (3) analyzing processes within your own organization (or health system) that are worthy of being emulated. In any of these three cases, the necessary analysis will rely on one or both of the following methods: parametric analysis or process analysis. In parametric analysis, the characteristics or attributes of similar services or products are examined. In process analysis, the process that serves as a standard for comparison is examined in detail to learn how and why it performs the way it does.

Benchmarking is used for opportunity assessment. Opportunity assessment, used for strategic planning and for process engineering, provides information about the way things should or possibly could be. Benchmarking is a primary information-gathering approach for opportunity assessment when it is used in this way.

Benchmarking in Health Care

Financial benchmarking compares financial measures among benchmarking groups. This is the most common type of "peer group" health care benchmarking in use. An example of a health care financial benchmarking report is provided in Table 12–6.

Table 12–6 Financial Benchmark Example

Indicator	Total	Upper Quartile	Mid-Quartile	Low Quartile
No. of hospitals	500.0	105.0	305.0	90.0
Total margin (%)	4.1	11.0	4.5	−6.0
Occupancy (%)	64.5	65.7	64.0	56.1
Deductions from GPR (%)	29.0	28.5	29.2	31.3
Medicare (%GPR)	53.0	55.1	52.2	50.4
Medicaid (%GPR)	10.0	8.4	9.7	13.7
Self-pay (%GPR)	7.0	8.5	7.1	6.4
Managed care plans (%GPR)*	16.0	13.0	17.0	17.5
Other third party (%GPR)	14.0	15.0	14.0	12.0
Outpatient revenue (%GPR)	22.0	25.0	21.8	17.7
No. of days in accounts receivable	75.0	70.0	74.0	80.0
Cash flow as a percentage of total debt	30.0	60.0	27.0	−0.5
Long-Term Debt as a Percentage of total assets	35.0	26.0	36.0	42.0
Change in admissions (1993–1997, %)	−7.0	−3.7	−6.3	−15.8
Change in inpatient days (1993–1997, %)	−6.0	−1.8	−6.5	−11.1

*Note: Managed care plans other than Title XVIII or Title XIX. All amounts are fictitious.

Source: Reprinted from J.J. Baker, *Activity-Based Costing and Activity-Based Management for Health Care,* p. 140, © 1998, Aspen Publishers, Inc.

The computation of ratios included in this report has been discussed in the preceding chapter. The computation of quartiles is described later in this chapter.

Statistical benchmarking is a related method of benchmarking. In this case, the statistics of utilization and service delivery, on which inflow and outflow are based, are compared with those of certain other hospitals.

In summary, benchmarking is a comparative method that allows an overview of the individual organization's indicators. Objective measurement criteria are always required for best practices purposes.

ECONOMIC MEASURES

Other performance measures may be made outside the actual confines of the facility. A good example of a widespread performance measure would be the role of community hospitals in the performance of local economies. Nonprofit organizations in particular are concerned about their ability to measure such performance. This case study gives a specific direction for such measurement efforts.

MEASUREMENT TOOLS

Pareto Analysis

Creating benchmarks, especially in an organization committed to continuous quality improvement, ultimately leads managers to exploring how to improve some step in a process. Pareto analysis is an analytical tool that employs the Pareto principle and helps in this exploration. Pareto was a 19th-century economist who was a pioneer in applying mathematics to economic theory. His Pareto principle states that 80 percent of an organization's problems, for example, are caused by 20 percent of the possible causes: thus the "80/20 Rule."

The usual way to display a Pareto analysis is through the construction of a Pareto diagram. A Pareto diagram displays the important causes of variation, as reflected in data collected on the causes of such variation. Figure 12–3 presents an example of a Pareto diagram. This example reinforces the idea behind the Pareto analysis: that the majority of problems are due to a small number of identifiable causes.

The chief financial officer of XYZZ Hospital believes that the billing and collection department is inefficient—or, to be more specific, that the process is probably inefficient. An activity analysis is conducted. It shows that billing personnel are spending much time on unproductive work. This Pareto diagram displays the activities involved in resubmitting denied bills. (Resubmitting denied bills is an inefficient and nonproductive activity, as we have discussed in a preceding chapter.)

Constructing a Pareto diagram is really simple. The first step is to prepare a table that shows the activities recorded, the numbers of times the activities were observed, and the percentage of the total number of times represented by each count. In Figure 12–3, the total number of times these activities were observed is 43. The number of times that processing denied bills for resubmission (coded as PDB) was observed is 22. Thus, $100 (22/43) = 51$ percent. Similar calculations complete the table. The table of observations is shown in its entirety within the figure.

The Pareto diagram has two vertical axes, the left one corresponding to the "No." column in the table, the right one corresponding to the "%" column in the table. On the horizontal axis, the activities are listed, creating bases of equal length for

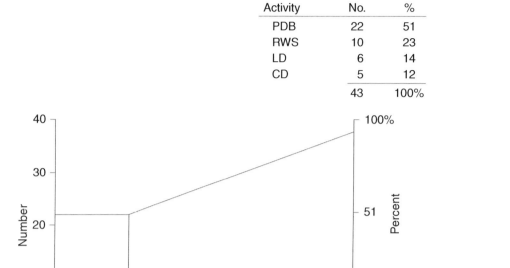

Activity	No.	%
PDB	22	51
RWS	10	23
LD	6	14
CD	5	12
	43	100%

Key to Activity Codes

PDB = Process Denied Bills
RWS = Review with Supervisor
LD = Locate Documentation
CD = Copy Documentation

Figure 12–3 Pareto Analysis of Billing Department Data.

the rectangles shown in the diagram. The activities are listed in decreasing order of occurrence. Constructing the diagram in this manner means that the most frequently observed activity lies on the left extreme of the diagram and the least frequently observed activity on the right extreme. The heights of the rectangles are drawn to show the frequencies of the activities, and then the sides of the rectangle are drawn.

The next step is to locate the cumulative percentage of the activities, using the right-hand axis. The cumulative percent for the first rectangle, labeled *PDB,* is 51 percent. (The calculation of the 51 percent was pre-

viously explained.) For the second rectangle from the left, labeled *RWS,* the cumulative percentage is 51 + 23 = 74 percent. The 74 percent is plotted over the right-hand side of the rectangle labeled *RWS.* The next cumulative percentage, for the third rectangle from the left, labeled *LD,* is 51 + 23 + 14 = 88 percent. The 88 percent is plotted over the right-hand side of the rectangle labeled *LD.* The last cumulative percentage is, of course, 100 percent (51 + 23 + 14 + 12 = 100 percent), and it is plotted over the right-hand side of the last rectangle on the right, labeled *CD.*

Now draw straight lines between the plotted cumulative percentages as shown in Exhibit 12–1. The next step is to label the axes and add a title to the diagram. In Figure 12–3, the tallest rectangle could be lightly shaded to highlight the most frequent activity, suggesting the one that may deserve first priority in problem solving.

In general, the activities requiring priority attention, the "vital few," will appear on the left of the diagram where the slope of the curve is steepest. Pareto diagrams are often constructed before and after improvement efforts for comparative purposes. When comparing before and after, if the improvement measures are effective, either the order of the bars will change or the curve will be much flatter.

In conclusion, note that many authorities recommend that Pareto analysis take the *costs* of the activities into account. The concern is that a very frequent problem may nevertheless imply less overall cost than a relatively rare but disastrous problem. Also, before basing a Pareto analysis on frequencies, as this example does, the analyst needs to decide that the seriousness of the problem is roughly proportional to the frequency. If seriousness fails to satisfy this criterion, then activities should be measured in some other way. Figure 12–3 underlines the importance of judging the relevance of the measurements used in a Pareto analysis.

Quartile Computation

Reporting by quartiles is an effective way to show ranges of either financial or statistical results. Quartiles represent a distribution into four classes, each of which contains one quarter of the whole. Each of the four classes is a quartile. Quartile computation is not very complicated, although several steps are involved. We can use the outpatient revenue line item in Table 12–6 to illustrate the computation of quartile data. (Outpatient revenue, expressed as a percentage of all revenue, is found on the tenth line down from the top in Table 12–6.) We see from the first line that 500 hospitals were in the group used for benchmarking. The median is found for the outpatient revenue of the entire group of hospitals. (Most computer spreadsheet programs offer median computation as an available function.) Then each hospital's revenue is identified as a percentage of this median. These percentages are arrayed. In the case of this report, cutoffs were then made to arrange the arrayed percentages into three groups. The percentages that were between 0 and 25 percent were designated as the low-quartile group. The percentages that were between 75 and 100 percent were designated as the high-quartile group. The percentages that were between 25 and 75 percent were designated as the mid-quartile group.

The average (also known as the arithmetic mean) of each quartile group is then presented in this report. Thus, the outpatient revenue (expressed as a percentage of gross revenue) for the upper-quartile group in the report is 25.0; for the middle-quartile group, 21.8; and for the low-quartile group, 17.7. (A grand total of the entire 500 hospitals is also computed and presented in the left-hand column; the grand total amounts to 22 percent.) In summary, quartiles are based on a quantitative method of computation and are an effective way to illustrate a variety of performance measures.

INFORMATION CHECKPOINT

What Is Needed?	An example of a staffing forecast created in your organization.
Where Is It Found?	In the files of the supervisor who is responsible for staffing.
How Is It Used?	Use the example to learn the nature of the assumptions that were used and the setup of the forecast itself.

 KEY TERMS

Benchmarking
Case Mix Adjusted
Common Sizing
Controllable Costs
Forecasts
Noncontrollable Costs
Pareto Analysis
Performance
Performance Measures
Quartiles
Trend Analysis
Vertical Analysis

 DISCUSSION QUESTIONS

1. Do any of the reports you receive in the course of your work use common sizing? If so, how is it used in your managerial reports?
2. Do any of the reports you work with use trend analysis? If so, how is trend analysis used in your reports?
3. Are you or your immediate supervisor involved with staffing decisions? If so, are you aware of how staffing forecasts are done in your organization? Describe an example.
4. Does your organization use measurements such as the case mix adjustment over time? If not, do you believe they should? Why?
5. Does your organization use financial benchmarking? Would you use it if you had a chance to do so? Why?

CHAPTER 13

Budgeting and Variance Analysis

PROGRESS NOTES

After completing this chapter, you should be able to

1. Understand the difference between static and flexible budgets.
2. Effectively review a budget.
3. Understand how to build a budget.
4. Perform budget variance analysis.

ciation's (AHA's) objectives for the budgeting process:

1. To provide a written expression, in quantitative terms, of a hospital's policies and plans
2. To provide a basis for the evaluation of financial performance in accordance with a hospital's policies and plans
3. To provide a useful tool for the control of costs
4. To create cost awareness throughout the organization[1]

Types of Budgets

Static Budget

A static budget is essentially based on a single level of operations. After a static budget has been approved and finalized, that single level of operations (volume) is never adjusted. Budgets are measured by how they differ from actual results. Thus, a variance is the difference between an actual result and a budgeted amount when the budgeted amount is a financial variable reported by the accounting system. The variance may or may not be a standard amount, and it may or may not be a benchmark amount.[2]

BUDGETS

A budget is an organization-wide instrument. The organization's objectives define the specific activities to be performed, how they will be assembled, and the particular levels of operation, whereas the organization's performance standards or norms set out the anticipated levels of individual performance. The budget is the instrument through which activities are quantified in financial terms.

A health care standard view of budgeting is illustrated by the American Hospital Asso-

The computation of a static budget variance only requires one calculation, as follows:

$$\begin{matrix} \text{Actual} \\ \text{Results} \end{matrix} - \begin{matrix} \text{Static Budget} \\ \text{Amount} \end{matrix} = \begin{matrix} \text{Static Budget} \\ \text{Variance} \end{matrix}$$

The basic thing to understand is that static budgeted expense amounts never change when volume actually changes during the year. In the case of health care, we can use patient days as an example of level of volume, or output. Assume that the budget anticipated 400,000 patient days this year (patient days equating to output of service delivery; thus, 400,000 output units). Further assume that the revenue was budgeted for the expected 400,000 patient days and that the expenses were also budgeted at an appropriate level for the expected 400,000 patient days. Now assume that only 360,000, or 90 percent, of the patient days are going to actually be achieved for the year. The budgeted revenues and expenses still reflect the original expectation of 400,000 patient days. This example is a static budget; it is geared toward only one level of activity, and the original level of activity remains constant or static.

Flexible Budget

A flexible budget is one that is created using budgeted revenue and/or budgeted cost amounts. A flexible budget is adjusted, or flexed, to the actual level of output achieved (or perhaps expected to be achieved) during the budget period.[3] A flexible budget thus looks toward a range of activity or volume (versus only one level in the static budget).

Flexible budgets became important to health care when diagnosis-related groups (DRGs) were established in hospitals in the 1980s. The development of a flexible budget requires more time and effort than does the development of a static budget. If the organization is budgeting with workload standards, for example, the static budget projects expenses at a single normative level of workload activity, whereas the flexible budget projects expenses at various levels of workload activity.[4]

The concept of the flexible budget addresses workloads, control, and planning. The budget checklists contained in Appendix A are especially applicable to the flexible budget approach.

Reviewing a Budget

The manager needs to know how to review a budget effectively. To do so, the manager needs to understand how the budget report format is constructed. In general, the usual operating expense budget that is under review will have a column for actual expenditures, a column for budgeted expenditures, and a column for the difference between the two. Usually, the actual expense column and the budget column will both have a vertical analysis of percentages (as discussed in the preceding chapter). Each difference line item will have a horizontal analysis (also discussed in the preceding chapter) that measures the amount of the difference against the budget. Table 13–1 illustrates the operating expense budget configuration just described. Notice that the "Difference" column has both positive and negative numbers in it (the negative numbers being set off with parentheses). Thus, the positive numbers indicate budget overage, such as the dietary line, which had an actual expense of $405,000 against a budget figure of $400,000, resulting in a $5,000 difference. The next line is maintenance. This department did not exceed its budget, so the difference is in parentheses; the maintenance budget amounted to

Table 13–1 Comparative Analysis of Budget versus Actual

	Hospital 1					
	Year 2 Actual		Year 2 Budget		Difference	
	$$	%	$$	%	$$	%
General services expense						
Dietary	$405,000	45	$400,000	46	$5,000	12.5
Maintenance	270,000	30	290,000	33	(20,000)	(6.9)
Laundry	45,000	5	50,000	6	(5,000)	(10.0)
Housekeeping	180,000	20	130,000	15	50,000	38.5
General Service expense	$900,000	100	$870,000	100	$30,000	3.5

$290,000, and actual expenses were only $270,000, so the $20,000 difference is in parentheses. In this case, parentheses are good (under budget) and no parentheses is bad (over budget).

Another computation the manager needs to know is how to annualize partial-year expenses. Table 13–2 sets out the actual 10-month expenses for the operating room. But these expenses are going to be compared against a 12-month budget. What to do? The actual 10-month expenses are converted, or annualized, to a 12-month basis, as shown in the second column of Table 13–2. These computations were performed on a computer spreadsheet; however, the calculation is as follows. Using the first line as an example, $50,431 is 10 months worth of expenses; therefore, one month's expense is one tenth of $50,431 or $5,043. To annualize for 12 months worth of expenses, the 10-month total of $50,431 is increased by two more months at $5,043 apiece (50,431 plus 5,043 plus 5,043 equals 60,517, the annualized figure).

Although we have used examples illustrating operating expenses, budgets can, of course, also include revenue. Whether the manager's budget will include revenue (or volume) will generally depend on whether the unit is a responsibility center (discussed in a previous chapter).

A checklist for reviewing a budget appears as Exhibit 13–1. The items are self-explanatory.

Building a Budget

Building a budget means making a series of assumptions. The budget process should begin with a review of strategy and objectives. Forecasting workload is a critical part of building a budget; the workload should tie into expected volume for the new budget period. Good information is necessary to forecast workload. For example, Table 13–3 presents total nursing hours by unit. But there is not enough detail in this report to use because it does not indicate, among other things, hours by type of staff and/or staff level. Sufficient information at the proper level of detail is essential in creating a budget.

Another critical assumption in building a budget is whether special projects are going to use resources during the new budget period. Still another factor to consider is whether operations are going to be placed

Table 13–2 Annualizing Operating Room Partial-Year Expenses

	Expenses	
Account	Actual 10 Month	Annualized 12 Month
Social Security	50,431	60,517
Pension	17,229	20,675
Health Insurance	7,018	8,422
Child Care	3,803	4,564
Patient Accounting	129,463	155,356
Admitting	91,878	110,254
Medical Records	76,432	91,718
Dietary	22,938	27,526
Medical Waste	1,981	2,377
Sterile Procedures	65,600	78,720
Laundry	33,911	40,693
Depreciation—Equipment	72,815	87,378
Depreciation—Building	34,481	41,377
Amortization—Interest	(4,849)	(5,819)
Insurance	3,513	4,216
Administration	48,305	57,966
Medical Staff	1,435	1,722
Community Relations	41,511	49,813
Materials Management	53,811	64,573
Human Resources	25,888	31,066
Nursing Administration	68,726	82,471
Data Processing	14,846	17,815
Fiscal	14,750	17,700
Telephone	2,366	2,839
Utilities	22,005	26,406
Plant	64,664	77,597
Environmental Services	27,395	32,874
Safety	1,680	2,016
Quality Management	8,347	10,016
Medical Staff	7,870	9,444
Continuous Quality Improvement	4,079	4,895
EE Health	474	569
Total Allocated	1,014,796	1,217,756
All Other Expenses	1,009,673	1,211,608
Total Expense	2,024,469	2,429,364

Source: Adapted from J.J. Baker, *Activity-Based Costing and Activity-Based Management for Health Care,* p. 190, © 1998, Aspen Publishers, Inc.

under some type of unusual or inconvenient circumstances during the new budget period. A good example would be renovation of the work area. Exhibit 13–2 sets out a series of questions and steps to undertake when commencing to build a budget.

To build a flexible budget that looks toward a range of volume, or activity, instead of a single static amount, one must first determine the relevant range of volume, or activity. Thus, the outer limits of fluctuations are determined by defining the relevant range. Next, one must analyze the patterns of the costs expected to occur during the budget period. Third, one must separate the costs by behavior (fixed or variable). Finally, one can prepare the flexible budget—

Exhibit 13–1 Checklist for Reviewing a Budget

1. Is this budget static (not adjusted for volume) or flexible (adjusted for volume during the year)?
2. Are the figures designated as fixed or variable?
3. Is the budget for a defined unit of authority?
4. Are the line items within the budget all expenses (and revenues, if applicable) that are controllable by the manager?
5. Is the format of the budget comparable with that of previous periods so that several reports over time can be compared if so desired?
6. Are actual and budget for the same period?
7. Are the figures annualized?
8. Test one line-item calculation. Is the math for the dollar difference computed correctly? Is the percentage properly computed based on a percentage of the budget figure?

Table 13–3 Nursing Hours Report

Unit		Nursing Hours	
No.	Description	Regular	Overtime
620	S-MED-SURG DIV 5	72,509	6,042
630	N-MED-SURG DIV B	40,248	3,354
640	N-MED SURG DIV D	42,182	3,515
645	N-INTENSIVE CARE UNIT	55,952	4,663
655	S-INTENSIVE CARE UNIT	52,000	4,333
660	S-SURG. ICU	21,840	1,820
665	S-STEPDOWN	52,208	4,351

a budget capable of projecting what costs will be incurred at different levels of volume, or activity.

VARIANCE ANALYSIS

This discussion assumes a flexible budget prepared in accordance with the steps just described. A variance is, basically, the difference between standard and actual prices and quantities. Variance analysis analyzes these differences. Flexible budgeting variance analysis was conceived by industry and subsequently discovered by health care. It provides a method to get more information about the composition of departmental expenses. The method subdivides total variance into three types:

1. *Volume variance.* The volume variance is the portion of the overall variance caused by a difference between the expected workload and the actual workload and is calculated as the difference between the total budgeted cost based on a predetermined, expected workload level and the amount that would have been budgeted had the actual workload been known in advance.[5]

Exhibit 13–2 Checklist for Building a Budget

1. What is the proposed volume for the new budget period?
2. What is the appropriate inflow (revenues) and outflow (cost of services delivered) relationship?
3. What will the appropriate dollar cost be?
   (Note: this question requires a series of assumptions about the nature of the operation for the new budget period.)
3a. Forecast service-related workload.
3b. Forecast non–service-related workload.
3c. Forecast special project workload if applicable.
3d. Coordinate assumptions for proportionate share of interdepartmental projects.
4. Will additional resources be available?
5. Will this budget accomplish the appropriate managerial objectives for the organization?

2. *Quantity (or use) variance.* The quantity variance is also known as the *use variance* or the *efficiency variance.* It is the portion of the overall variance that is caused by a difference between the budgeted and actual quantity of input needed per unit of output and is calculated as the difference between the actual quantity of inputs used per unit of output multiplied by the actual output level and the budgeted unit price.
3. *Price (or spending) variance.* The price variance is also known as the *spending* or *rate variance.* This variance is the portion of the overall variance caused by a difference between the actual and expected price of an input and is calculated as the difference between

the actual and budgeted unit price or hourly rate multiplied by the actual quantity of goods or labor consumed per unit of output and by the actual output level.

Variance analysis can be performed as a two- or a three-variance analysis. (There is also a five-variance analysis that is beyond the scope of this discussion.) The two-variance analysis involves the volume variance as compared with budgeted costs (defined as standard hours for actual production). The three-variance analysis involves the three types of variances defined above. Figure 13–1 illustrates these components.

The makeup of the two variance is compared with the three variance in Figure 13–2. As is shown, two elements (A and B) remain the same in both methods. The third element (C) is a single amount in the two-variance method but splits into two amounts (C-1 and C-2) in the three-variance method.

Actual computation is illustrated in Figure 13–3 for two-variance analysis and Figure 13–4 for three-variance analysis. The A, B, C, C-1, and C-2 designations are carried

forward from Figure 13–2. In Figure 13–3, the two-variance calculation is illustrated, and a proof total computation is supplied at the bottom of the illustration. In Figure 13–4, the three-variance calculation is likewise illustrated, and a proof total computation is also supplied at the bottom of the illustration. This set of three illustrations deserves study. If the manager understands the concept presented here, then he or she understands the theory of variance analysis.

Another oddity in variance analysis that contributes to confusion is this. All three variable cost elements—that is, direct materials, direct labor, and variable overhead—can have a price variance and a quantity variance computed. But the variance is not known by the same name in all instances. Exhibit 13–3 sets out the different names. Even though the names differ, the calculation for all three is the same. Note, too, that variance analysis is primarily a matter of input–output analysis. The inputs represent actual quantities of direct materials, direct labor, and variable overhead used. The outputs represent the services or products delivered (e.g., produced) for the applicable time period, expressed in terms of standard

	Elements of Two-Variance Analysis		Elements of Three-Variance Analysis
1	Volume Variance (Activity Variance)	**1**	Volume Variance (Activity Variance)
2	Budget Variance	**2**	Quantity Variance (Use Variance, Efficiency Variance)
		3	Price Variance (Spending Variance, Rate Variance)

Figure 13–1 Elements of Variance Analysis. Courtesy of Resource Group, Ltd., Dallas, Texas.

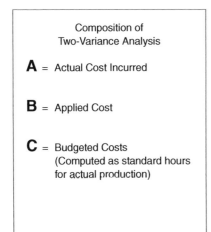
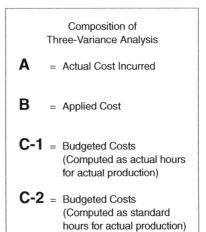

Figure 13–2 Composition of Two- and Three-Variance Analysis. Courtesy of Resource Group, Ltd., Dallas, Texas.

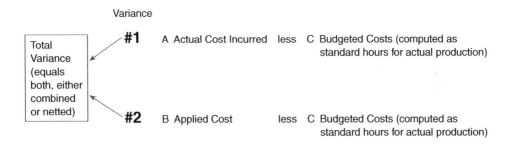

Note: To obtain proof total, perform the following calculation:
A, Actual Cost Incurred, less B, Applied Cost = Total Variance

Figure 13–3 A Calculation of Two-Variance Analysis. Courtesy of Resource Group, Ltd., Dallas, Texas.

quantity (in the case of materials) or of standard hours (in the case of labor). In other words, the standard quantity or standard hours equates to what should have been used (the standard) rather than what was actually used. This is an important point to remember.

Example of Variance Analysis

An example of variance analysis in a hospital system is given in Exhibit 13–4. It deals with price or spending variance and quantity or use variance. The price variance is expressed in RVUs. The quantity variance is

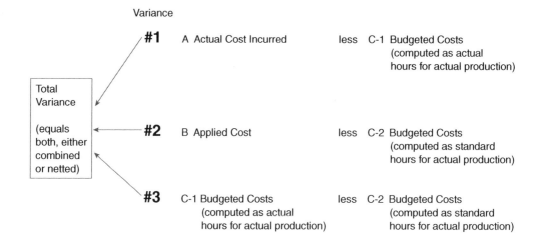

Figure 13–4 Calculation of Three-Variance Analysis. Courtesy of Resource Group, Ltd., Dallas, Texas.

Exhibit 13–3 Different Names for Materials, Labor, and Overhead Variances

Price or Spending Variance = Materials Price Variance	[for direct materials]
Price or Spending Variance = Labor Rate Variance	[for direct labor]
Price or Spending Variance = Overhead Spending Variance	[for variable overhead]

broken out into four subtypes—patient, caregiver, environmental, and efficiency variances, all of which are expressed in RVUs. Finally, it is assumed that the budgeted activity level is equal to the standard activity level for purposes of this example.

The flexible budget calculation ($2,885,989) is based on actual quantity. When the $2,885,989 is compared with the actual cost of $2,661,523 for this activity center, a favorable price variance of $224,466 is realized. When the $2,885,989 is compared with the budgeted cost of $2,700,000 for this activity center, an unfavorable quantity variance of ($185,989) is realized.

In closing, when should variances be investigated? Variances will fluctuate within some type of normal range. The trick is to separate normal randomness from those factors requiring correction. The manager would be well advised to calculate the cost–benefit of performing a variance analysis before commencing the analysis.

Exhibit 13–4 St. Joseph Hospital Nursing Center Variance Analysis

Summary Variance Report for Nursing Activity Center

Actual Costs	Flexible Budget (based on actual quantity)	Budgeted Costs
641,331 RVUs × $4.15 per RVU = $2,661,523	641,331 RVUs × $4.50 per RVU = $2,885,989	600,000 RVUs × $4.50 per RVU = $2,700,000

Price Variance	Quantity Variance
= $224,466* (favorable)	= $185,989[†] (unfavorable)

Assume the following information for the nursing activity center of St. Joseph Hospital for the month of September:

Input Data
Nursing Activity Center
Cost Driver = Number of Relative Value Units (RVUs)

Actual	Budget
Activity Level = 641,331 RVUs	Activity Level = 600,000 RVUs
Overhead Costs = $2,661,523	Overhead Costs = $2,700,000
Actual Cost per RVU = $4.15	Budgeted Cost per RVU = $4.50

*2,885,989 < 2,661,523 > = 224,466
[†]2,885,989 < 2,700,000 > 185,989.
Source: Adapted from S. Upda, Activity-Based Costing for Hospitals, *Health Care Management Review,* Vol. 21, No. 3, p. 93, © 1996, Aspen Publishers, Inc.

   INFORMATION CHECKPOINT

What Is Needed?	Example of variance analysis performed on a budget.
Where Is It Found?	Possibly with the supervisor responsible for the budget. More likely it will be found in the office of the strategic planner or financial analyst charged with actually performing the analysis.
How Is It Used?	To find where and how variances have occurred during the budget period, in order to manage better in the future.

KEY TERMS

Budget
Flexible Budget
Static Budget
Three-Variance Method
Two-Variance Method
Variance Analysis

 DISCUSSION QUESTIONS

1. Do you believe your organization uses a flexible or static budget? Why do you think so?
2. If you reviewed a budget at your workplace, do you think the major increases and decreases could be explained?
3. If so, why? If not, why not?
4. Do you believe variance analysis (or a better variance analysis) would be a good idea at your workplace? If so, why?

CHAPTER 14

Capital Expenditure Budgets

PROGRESS NOTES

After completing this chapter you should be able to

1. Recognize the reason that a capital expenditure budget is necessary.
2. Review the cash flow and the startup cost concept.
3. Understand differences between cash flow reporting methods.
4. Recognize types of capital expenditure budget proposals.
5. Understand about evaluating capital expenditure proposals.

OVERVIEW

Capital expenditures involve the acquisition of assets that are long lasting, such as equipment, buildings, and land. Therefore, capital expenditure budgets are usually intended to plan, monitor, and control long-term financial issues. Decisions must be made about the future use of funds in order to complete these types of budgets.

Operations budgets, on the other hand, generally deal with actual short-term revenues and expenses necessary to operate the facility. For example, the Great Shores Health System's operations budgets may usually be created to cover the next year only (a 12-month period), while Great Shores capital expenditure budgets may be created to cover a five-year span (a 60-month period) or even a ten-year span.

It is also important to note that the budget for capital expenditures is usually part of an overall, or comprehensive, financial budget. Responsibility for the comprehensive financial budget always rests with upper-level financial officers of the organization and is beyond the scope of this chapter.

CREATING THE CAPITAL EXPENDITURE BUDGET

The capital expenditure budget, which may sometimes be identified by another name, such as "capital spending plan," usually consists two parts. The first part of the budget represents spending for capital assets that have already been acquired and are in place. This spending protects an existing asset; you are essentially spending in order to protect that which you already have. The second part of the budget represents spending for new capital assets. In this case, you will be expending capital funds to acquire new assets such as equipment, buildings, and land.

The "existing asset" part of the budget forces planning questions about whether existing equipment and buildings should be kept in their present condition (which can involve repair and maintenance expenses), renovated, or replaced. Renovating equipment or buildings implies a large expenditure that would be capitalized. (To be capitalized means the expenditure would be placed on the balance sheet as an additional capital cost that is recognized as an asset.)

The "new capital asset" part of the budget forces more planning questions. In this case, the questions are about new assets. The reasons for new asset spending may involve:

- Expansion of capacity in a department or program
- Creation of a new facility, department, or program
- New equipment to improve productivity
- New equipment or space to comply with federal or state requirements

It should also be noted that acquiring new assets results in additional capital costs that will be placed on the balance sheet as assets. For more information, refer to Chapter 3.

BUDGET CONSTRUCTION TOOLS

How the capital expenditure budget is constructed may be predetermined by requirements of the organization. Your facility or practice may have a template that must be used. This takes the decision out of your hands. Otherwise, you will have to decide which tool or tools will be most effective to build your capital expenditure budget.

One important tool is net cash flow reporting. The concept of cash flow analysis, usually an important part of the capital expenditure budget, is described later here. But how will the cash flow be reported? Four methods are discussed in this section.

Cash Flow Concept

As its title implies, a cash flow analysis illustrates how the project's cash is expected to move over a period of time. Many analyses concentrate only on the cash expenditure for the equipment. (This is, after all, a "capital expenditure" budget.) Other analyses, however, will also take revenue earned into account.

In any case, it is always important to report the net cash flow. While most line items will usually be expenditures, called cash outflow, sometimes there will also be cash receipts, called cash inflow. For example, if a new piece of equipment will replace an old one, and the old replaced equipment will be sold for cash, the cash received from the sale will represent a cash receipt.

Cash flow must also be reported as cumulative. This means the accumulated effect of cash inflows and cash outflows must be added and/or subtracted to show the overall net accumulated result. In our example mentioned previously here where the old equipment might be sold, the cumulative cash flow is illustrated in Table 14–1. As you can see, the initial expenditure or cash spent (outflow) is decreased by the cash received (inflow) to produce a net cumulative result.

Cash Flow Reporting Methods

Cash flow is typically reported using one of four methods. They include:

Table 14–1 Ilustration of Cumulative Cash Flow

Line Number		XCash Spent (Outflow)	Cash Received (Inflow)	Cumulative Cash Flow
1	Buy new equipment	(50,000)	—	(50,000)
2	Sell old equipment that is being replaced	—	+ 6,000	(44,000)

- Payback method
- Accounting rate of return
- Net present value
- Internal rate of return

A previous chapter of this book has explained and illustrated each of the four methods. Their advantages and disadvantages for purposes of capital expenditure budgeting are summarized later here.

Payback Method

The payback method is based on cash flow. This method recognizes the cash flows that are necessary to recover the initial cash invested. The payback method is advantageous because it is easy to understand and highlights risks. However, it does not take either profitability or the time value of money into account.

Accounting Rate of Return

The accounting rate of return is based on profitability. However, it does not take the time value of money into account.

Net Present Value

Net present value, or NPV, is a discounted cash flow method. It is based on cash flows in that it takes all the cash (incoming and outgoing) into account over the life of the equipment (or, if applicable, over the life of the relevant project). Although the NPB is based on cash flows, it also takes profitability and the time value of money into account.

Internal Rate of Return

Internal rate of return, or IRR, is also a discounted cash flow method that takes all incoming and outgoing cash into account over the life of the equipment (or the project). It, too, takes profitability and the time value of money into account.

The use of net present value, the internal rate of return, and so forth is the vocabulary of capital budgeting. It is also an important part of the language of finance. Therefore, it is important to understand the differences between the four methods. Review Chapter 11 for more detail. Chapter 16 presents a step-by-step method for net present value computation that assists in this understanding.

Startup Cost Concept

If the proposal for capital expenditures incorporates operational expenses, the concept of startup costs must also be taken into consideration. In these cases, management believes the cost of starting up a new service line or a new program should be included as part of the original investment. Although such operational costs do not fall into a strict definition of capital expenditure budgeting, the requirement is common enough to warrant discussion.

FUNDING REQUESTS

This section discusses the process of requesting capital expenditure funds and the types of proposals that might be submitted for consideration.

The Process of Requesting Capital Expenditure Funds

Different departments or divisions often have to compete for capital expenditure funding. The hospital's radiology department director may want new equipment, but so does the surgery department director, and so on. The various requests for funding are often collected and subjected to a review process in order to make decisions about where and to whom the available capital expenditure funds will go. While the upper levels of management make overall decisions about future use of funds, the departmental funding requests represent the first step in the overall process.

The process involved for capital expenditure funding requests varies according to the organization. Size plays a part. We would expect a giant hospital to have a more complex process than, say, a two-doctor physician practice, due to its sheer size. The corporate culture of the organization plays a part, too. Some organizations are extremely structured, while others are flexible in their management principles. And in some facilities, politics may also be a part in the process of making and reviewing funding requests.

Types of Capital Expenditure Proposals

The type of proposal affects its size and scope. Proposal types commonly include the following types of requests:

- Acquiring new equipment
- Upgrading existing equipment
- Replacing existing equipment with new equipment
- Funding new programs
- Funding expansion of existing programs
- Acquiring capital assets for future use

Certain of these types may sometimes be paired as either/or choices in capital expenditure proposals. All six types of proposals are discussed in this section.

Acquiring New Equipment

The reason why new equipment is needed must be clearly stated. The acquisition cost must be a reasonable figure that contains all appropriate specifications. The number of years of useful life that can be reasonably expected from the equipment is also an important assumption.

Upgrading Existing Equipment

The reason why an upgrade is necessary must be clearly stated. What is the impact? What will the outcomes be from the upgrade? The upgrade costs must be a reasonable figure that also contains all appropriate specifications. Will the upgrade extend the useful life of the equipment? If so, by how long?

Replacing Existing Equipment with New Equipment

The rationale for replacing existing equipment with new equipment must be clearly stated. Often a comparison may be made between upgrading and replacement in order to make a more compelling argument. The usual arguments in these comparisons revolve around improvements in technology in the new equipment that are more advanced than available upgrades to the old equipment. A favorite argument in favor of the new equipment is increased productivity and/or outcomes.

Funding New Programs

A proposal for new program capital expenditures must take startup costs into account. This type of proposal will generally be more extensive than a straightforward equipment replacement proposal because it involves a new venture without a previous history or proven outcomes.

Funding Expansion of Existing Programs

A proposal for expansion of an existing program is generally easier to prepare than a proposal for a new program. You will have statistics available from the existing program with which to make your arguments. In addition, any startup costs should be negligible for the existing program. The most difficult selling point may be comparison with other departments' funding requests.

Acquiring Capital Assets for Future Use

This type of proposal may be the most difficult to accomplish. Capital expenditures for future long-term use are often postponed by decision makers in cash-strapped organizations who must first fulfill immediate demands for funding. Consider, for example, a metropolitan hospital that is hemmed in on all sides by privately owned property. The hospital will clearly need expansion space in the future. An adjacent privately owned property comes on the market at a price less than its appraised value. Even through the expansion is not scheduled until several years in the future, it would be wise to seriously consider this acquisition of a capital asset for future use.

EVALUATING CAPITAL EXPENDITURE PROPOSALS

Management planning must involve the allocation of available financial resources for projects that promise to reap returns in the future. This applies to both for-profit and not-for-profit organizations.

Hard Choices: Rationing Available Capital

Most businesses, including those providing health care services and products, have only a limited amount of capital available for purposes of capital expenditure. It usually becomes necessary, then, to ration the available capital funds. Different organizations approach the rationing process in different ways. However, most organizations will consider the following factors in some fashion or other:

- Necessity for the request
- Cost of capital to the organization
- Return that could be realized on alternative investments

These three factors will probably be considered in a descending sequence of decision making. The overriding question is necessity. Necessity for the request pertains to the criticality of the need. What are the basic reasons for contemplating the capital expenditure? Are these reasons necessary? If so, how necessary?

While necessity is an overarching consideration, the cost of capital to the organization for the proposed capital expenditure is a computation of the sort we have previously discussed in this section. Although the answer to "what is the cost of capital" is provided in the form of a computation, the amount of the answer depends on the method selected to illustrate this cost.

The third element in management's decision-making sequence is what return could be realized on alternative investments of the available capital. This concept is known as "opportunity cost." The term is appropriate. Assume a rationing situation where unlimited funds are not available. Thus, when a choice is made to expend funds on capital project A, an opportunity is lost to expend those same funds on project B or project C. The choice of A thus costs the opportunity to gain benefits from B or C.

To summarize, the decision makers must apply judgment in making all these choices. Thus, the rationing of available capital becomes somewhat of a management art as well as a science.

The Review and Evaluation Process

The degree of attention paid to evaluation and the level of management responsible for making the decisions may be dictated by the overall availability of capital funding and by the amount of funds requested. Evalua-

tion of capital expenditure budget proposals may be objective or subjective. An impartial review process is most desirable.

An objective method usually involves scoring and/or ranking the competing proposals. In scoring, the basic approach generally focuses on a single proposal and evaluates it on a fixed set of criteria. In ranking, the proposal is compared with other proposals and ranked in accordance with a looser set of criteria.

The objective review and evaluation may actually first involve scoring to eliminate the very low-scoring proposals. The remaining higher scoring proposals may then be ranked in accordance with still another set of criteria.

The criteria may use may, in turn, contain quantitative items such as outcomes and/or productivity and may also contain qualitative items such as whether the proposal is in accordance with the organization's core mission.

Finally, some authorities believe the source of financing the project (whether it is internal or external, for example) should not be relevant to the investment decision. Real-world management, however, has a different view. How the project will be financed may be their first question in the review and evaluation process.

 INFORMATION CHECKPOINT

What Is Needed?	An example of an entire capital expenditure budget or a capital expenditure proposal for a particular project or a specific piece of equipment.
Where Is It Found?	Probably with your manager or the director of your department or, depending on the dollar amount proposed, perhaps with someone in the finance department.
How Is It Used?	The use would probably be one time. Can you tell if this is so?

KEY TERMS

Accounting Rate of Return
Capital Budget
Capitalized Asset
Cash Flow Analysis
Cumulative Cash Flow
Internal Rate of Return
Net Present Value
Operations Budget
Opportunity Cost
Payback Method
Unadjusted Rated of Return

 DISCUSSION QUESTIONS

1. Have you ever been involved in helping to create any part of a capital expenditure budget?
2. If so, which type of proposal was it? Was the proposal successful?
3. Do you recall whether any of the four cash flow reporting methods were used? If so, which one? Do you now think that was the best choice for the particular proposal?
4. If you were assigned to prepare a capital expenditure budget request, what two people would you most want to have on your team? Why? How would you expect to use them

A Further Discussion of Capital Budgeting Methods

This appendix presents a further discussion of the four methods of capital budgeting computations presented in Chapter 14.

ASSUMPTIONS

Item: Assume the purchase of a new piece of laboratory equipment is proposed.

Cost: The laboratory equipment will cost $70,000.

Useful life: It will last five years.

Remaining value (salvage value): The lab equipment will be sold for $10,000 (its salvage value) at the end of the five years.

Cost of capital: The estimated cost of capital for the hospital is ten percent.

Cash flow: The addition of this new piece of equipment is expected to generate additional revenue. In fact, the increase of revenue over expenses is expected to amount to $20,000 per year for the five years. The cash flow is therefore expected to be as follows: Year 0 = ($70,000); year 1 = $20,000; year 2 = $20,000; year 3 = $20,000; year 4 = $20,000; year 5 = $20,000. Note that year 0 is a negative figure and years 1 through 5 are positive figures.

PAYBACK METHOD

The payback method calculates how many periods are needed to recover the equipment's initial investment of $70,000. In this case the periods to be counted are years; thus there are five years, or five periods as shown in Table 14-A-1.

The investment of $70,000 is recovered half-way between year 3 and year 4, when the remaining balance to be recovered equals zero. Therefore the payback period is three and one-half years, expressed as 3.5 years.

Commentary: The payback method recognizes the cash flows that are necessary to recover the initial cash invested. The payback

Table 14–A–1 Payback Method Input

Year	Cash Flow	Balance
0	(70,000)	(70,000)
1	20,000	(50,000)
2	20,000	(30,000)
3	20,000	(10,000)
4	20,000	10,000
5	20,000	30,000

method is advantageous because it is easy to understand and highlights risks. However, it does not take either profitability or the time value of money into account.

UNADJUSTED RATE OF RETURN (AKA ACCOUNTANT'S RATE OF RETURN)

The unadjusted, or accountant's, rate of return is based on averages. The average accounting income is divided by the average level of investment to arrive at the accounting rate of return. Step One computes the average accounting income; Step Two computes the average level of investment, and Step Three then calculates the accounting rate of return.

Step 1: In this example the average accounting income is calculated by deducting depreciation (a non-cash amount) from the annual cash flow.

Step 1.1 First we must calculate the annual depreciation amount. In this example the depreciation is computed on a straight-line basis, which means the total amount of depreciation will equal the equipment's cost minus its salvage value.

The equipment's cost is $70,000 and its salvage value at the end of its five-year life is estimated to be $10,000. Therefore the total amount to be depreciated is the difference, or $60,000. To arrive at annual depreciation, the $60,000 is divided by the number of years of useful life, which is five years in this example. Therefore the annual amount of depreciation is $60,000 divided by five years, or $12,000 per year.

Step 1.2 Next we must use the depreciation amount to calculate the accounting income

per year. In this example the accounting income represents the cash flow per year of $20,000 as previously computed less the depreciation expense per year of $12,000. The remaining balance net of depreciation is $8,000 as shown in Table 14-A-2.

Step 2: In this example the average level of investment is determined by calculating the average investment represented by the equipment. We determine the average investment by computing its mid-point as follows.

Step 2.1 Determine the total investment by adding the initial investment of $70,000 and the salvage value of $10,000, for a total of $80,000.

Step 2.2 Now divide the total investment of $80,000 by 2. The answer of $40,000 indicates the mid-point of the investment and is considered the average investment over the five-year period of its useful life.

Step 3: The unadjusted or accounting rate of return is now calculated by dividing the average income (step 1) by the average investment (step 2). In this example, the unadjusted or accounting rate of return amounts to $8,0000 average income divided by $40,000 average investment, or a 20 percent rate of return.

Table 14–A–2 Accounting Income Input

Year	Cash Flow	Less Depreciation	Balance Net of Depreciation
1	20,000	12,000	8,000
2	20,000	12,000	8,000
3	20,000	12,000	8,000
4	20,000	12,000	8,000
5	20,000	12,000	8,000

Commentary: While the accounting rate of return is based on profitability, it does not take the time value of money into account. That is why it is known as the "unadjusted" rate of return. This method is used by many capital expenditure budget decision-makers.

NET PRESENT VALUE

Net present value, or NPV, is a discounted cash flow method. It is based on cash flows in that it takes all the cash (incoming and outgoing) into account over the life of the equipment. Table 14-A-3 shows the individual steps involved in the computation as follows.

Step 1: Enter the net cash flow on the table. (For this example, the net cash flow has already been calculated; see the middle column of Table 14-A-1. Also enter the salvage value.)

Step 2: Determine the cost of capital (which is 10% in this example). Look up the present value factor for 10% for each period. Also include the present value factor for the salvage value.

Step 3: Multiply the present value factor for each period times the net cash flow.

Step 4: Compute the net present value by first adding the present value answers for each operating period (Years 1 through 5 plus the salvage value) and then by subtracting the initial cash expenditure of $70,000 in Year 0 from the sum of the present value computations. In this example 70,000 is subtracted from a total of 81,980 to arrive at the net present value of $11,980 as shown in Table 14-A-3.

Commentary: Net present value takes all the cash (incoming and outgoing) into account over the life of the equipment. Even though the net present value is based on cash flow, it also takes profitability and the time value of money into account.

INTERNAL RATE OF RETURN

Internal rate of return, or IRR, computes the actual rate of return that is expected, or assumed, from an investment. The internal rate of return reflects the discount rate at which the investment's net present value equals zero.

The IRR computation will be compared against the cost of capital. In our example the cost of capital is 10%, as set out in our initial assumptions.

The internal rate of return or IRR seeks the rate of return that allows the net present value of the project to equal zero. The IRR expresses the rate of return that the organi-

Table 14–A–3 Net Present Value Computations

	Year 0	Year 1	Year 2	Year 3	Year 4	Year 5	Salvage Value
Net Cash Flow	(70,000)	20,000	20,000	20,000	20,000	20,000	10,000
Present value factor (10% cost of capital)	n/a	0.909	0.826	0.751	0.683	0.620	0.620
Present value answers	(70,000)	18,180	16,520	15,020	13,660	12,400	6,200
Net present value = 11,980							

zation can expect to earn when investing in the equipment (or the project, as the case may be).

The actual rate of return is determined by trial and error. The authorities say to "guess" and work forward from your initial "guess." An easier method to arrive at IRR is to use a business calculator and let it perform the computation for you. It is cumbersome but possible to arrive at the appropriate IRR by hand. An example follows.

This example solves for an initial investment of 70,000 and a positive cash flow of 20,000 per year for five years. Because the annual amount of 20,000 is the same for each of the five years, we can use the "Present Value of an Annuity of $1" presented in Appendix 11-C for this purpose.

The computation is approached in two steps as follows.

Step 1: initial investment (70,000) divided by the annual net cash inflow (20,000) equals the annuity present value (PV) factor for five periods. We compute 70,000 divided by 20,000 and arrive at a PV factor of 3.5.

Step 2: Now we refer to Appendix 11-C, the "Present Value of an Annuity of $1". We look across the "5" row (because that is the number of periods in our example). We are looking for the column that most closely resembles out PV factor of 3.5. On our table we find 3.605 in the 12% column and 3.433 in the 14% column. Obviously 3.5 will fall somewhere between these amounts. To find what 15% would be, we add the 3.605 to the 3.433 and divided by 2. The answer is 3.519 (3.605 + 3.433 = 7.038; 7.038 divided by 2 – 3.519). Thus we have found, by trial and error, that the rate of return in our example is approximately 15%.

As we have previously stated, an easier method to arrive at IRR is to use a business calculator and let it perform the computation for you. The business calculator will quickly give you a precise answer.

Many capital expenditure budget proposals also compare the rate of return to the organization's cost of capital. In our example the cost of capital is 10%, so the 15% IRR is clearly greater.

Commentary: Internal rate of return, or IRR, is also a discounted cash flow method that takes all incoming and outgoing cash into account over the life of the equipment (or the project). It, too, takes profitability and the time value of money into account.

PART VI

Allocate Resources and Acquire Funds

CHAPTER 15

Business Loans and Financing Costs

PROGRESS NOTES

After completing this chapter you should be able to

1. Understand what capital structure means.
2. Recognize four sources of capital.
3. Explain an amortization schedule.
4. Understand loan costs.

Business loans, as the term implies, represent debts incurred to assist in running a business. Whether to take on debt and how much to take on are common and necessary parts of financial planning. This type of planning involves the organization's capital structure, as discussed in the following section.

OVERVIEW OF CAPITAL STRUCTURE

"Capital" represents the financial resources of the organization and is generally considered to be a combination of debt and equity.

"Capital structure" means the proportion of debt versus equity within the organization. The phrase "capital structure" actually refers to the debt–equity relationship. For example, if a physician practice partnership owed $500,000 in debt and also had $500,000 in partner's equity, the partnership capital structure, or debt–equity relationship, would be 50–50.

Different industries typically have different debt–equity relationships. In the case of health care, the chief financial officer of the organization is usually responsible for guiding decisions about the proportion of debt. The chief financial officer will take into account various sources of capital, as discussed in the next section.

SOURCES OF CAPITAL

Sources of capital traditionally include four methods of obtaining funds:

- Borrowing from a lending institution
- Borrowing from investors
- Retaining the excess of revenues over expenses
- Selling an additional interest in the organization

Borrowing from a lending institution is generally classified by the length of the

149

loan. Short-term borrowing is commonly expected to be repaid within a twelve-month period. Long-term borrowing is usually to finance land, buildings, and/or equipment. Long-term borrowing for these purposes is usually accomplished by obtaining a mortgage from the lending institution.

Borrowing from investors assumes the organization is big enough and has the proper legal structure to do so. A common example of borrowing from investors is that of selling bonds. Bonds represent the company's promise to pay at a future date. When bonds are sold, the purchaser expects to receive a certain amount of annual interest and also expects that the bonds will be redeemed on a certain date, several years in the future.

Retaining the excess of revenues over expenses represents retaining operating profits to a proprietary, or for-profit, company. (Of course, this assumes there is an excess of funds to retain.) A not-for-profit organization may be bound by legal limitations on the retention of its funds. However, the not-for-profit organization can also sometimes rely on a different income stream. Church-affiliated not-for-profits, for example, may be able to solicit donations. This example represents a unique method of raising capital.

Selling an additional interest in the organization depends on its legal structure. Typically, this method involves a for-profit corporation selling additional shares of common stock to raise funds. Not-for-profit organizations are bound by legal limitations and may not be able to follow this route.

THE COSTS OF FINANCING

Financing costs typically involve interest expense and usually also involve loan costs, as described in this section.

Interest Expense

Payments on a business loan typically consist of two parts: principal and interest expense. The principal portion of the loan reduces the loan itself, while the rest of the payment is made up of interest on the remaining balance due on the loan.

The amount of principal and the amount of interest contained in each payment are illustrated in an "amortization schedule." For example, assume the purchase of equipment for $60,000. Monthly payments will be made over a three year period, and the annual, or per-year, interest rate will be 12 percent. The first six months of the amortization schedule for this loan is illustrated in Table 15–1. The entire 36-month amortization schedule is found in Appendix 15–A at the end of this chapter.

The interest expense for each monthly payment is computed on the principal balance remaining after the principal portion of the previous payment has been subtracted. The "Remaining Principal Balance" column shows the declining balance of the principal. Now refer to the "Remaining Principal Balance" column and compare it with the "Interest Portion of Payment" column. Remember that the 12 percent annual interest rate in this example amounts to one percent per month. You can see how ten percent of $60,000.00 amounts to a $600.00 interest payment for month 1; ten percent of $58,607.14 amounts to a $586.07 interest payment for month 2; and so on. The remainder of the payment amount—after interest expense—is then deducted from the principal amount due, as shown in Table 15–1. Thus, of the $1992.86 monthly payment 1, if $600.00 is interest, then $1,392.86 is the principal portion, and of the $1992.86 monthly payment 2, if $586.07 is interest,

Table 15–1 Loan Amortization Schedule

Payment Number	Total Payment	Principal Portion of Payment	Interest Expense Portion of Payment	Remaining Principal Balance
Beginning balance = 60,000.00				
1	1992.86	1392.86	600.00	58607.14
2	1992.86	1406.79	586.07	57200.35
3	1992.86	1435.07	572.00	55779.49
4	1992.86	1449.42	557.79	54344.42
5	1992.86	1463.91	543.44	52895.00
6	1992.86	1478.55	528.95	51431.09

then $1,406.79 is the principal portion, and so on.

Not all amortization schedules are set up in the same configuration. The columns that are shown can vary. For example, the entire 36-month amortization schedule for the Table 15–1 loan is contained in Appendix 15–A. Refer to this Appendix to see how the columns are different from Table 15–1. While the basic information necessary for computation is shown, the layout of the schedule is different.

Loan Costs

The term "loan costs" covers expenses necessary to close the loan. Loan closing costs generally include some expenses that would be reported in the current year and some other expenses that should be spread over several years.

Suppose, for example, the Great Lakes Home Health Agency bought a tract of land for expansion purposes. The home health agency paid a 20 percent down payment and obtained mortgage financing from a local bank for the remainder of the purchase price. When the loan was closed, meaning the transaction was completed, the statement that lists closing costs included prorated real estate taxes and "points" on the loan. Point represent a certain percentage of the loan amount paid, in this case to the bank, to cover costs of the financing.

The prorated real estate taxes represent an expense to be reported in the current year by the HHA. The points, however, would be spread over several years. How would this multiple-year reporting be handled? The total would first be placed on the balance sheet as an amount not yet recognized as expense. Each year a certain portion of that amount would be charged to current operations as an "amortized expense." Amortization expense is a noncash expense that is assigned to multiple reporting periods. It works much the same way as depreciation expense.

MANAGEMENT DECISIONS ABOUT BUSINESS LOANS

Decisions concerning how to obtain capital are an important part of financial management decision making. The chapter on capital expenditures discussed how new capital often has to be rationed within an organization. Repaying long-term loan obligations will impact the facility's cash flow for years to come, and decisions to undertake a large debt load should not be made lightly. Therefore, most institutions and/or companies have put a formal approval process into place that generally begins with the chief fi-nancial officer and his or her staff and pro-gresses upward all the way to board of trustee's approval, depending on the amount of the debt proposed.

Because of the implications, manage-ment decisions about business loans are often interwoven with strategic planning.

INFORMATION CHECKPOINT

What Is Needed?	An example of the details of a loan.
Where Is It Found?	In the department responsible for the organization's fi-nances.
How Is It Used?	Loan information is used by your financial decision makers.

KEY TERMS

Amortization Schedule
Bonds
Capital
Capital Structure
Equity Radio
Loan Costs
Long-Term Borrowing
Short-Term Borrowing

DISCUSSION QUESTIONS

1. Have you ever been informed of details about business loans in your unit or division?
2. If so, did you receive the information in the context of a new project (a new business loan that was made for purposes of the new project)?
3. Do the operating reports you receive contain information about loan costs, such as interest expense?
4. If so, do you think the interest expense seems reasonable for the operation? Why?

Sample Amortization Schedule

Principal borrowed: $60,000.00

Annual payments: 12

Total payments: 36

Annual interest rate: 12.00 percent

Periodic interest rate: 1.0000 percent

Regular payment amount: $1,992.86

Final balloon payment: $0.00

The following results are estimates that do not account for values being rounded to the nearest cent. See the amortization schedule for more accurate values.

Total repaid: $71,742.96
Total interest paid: $11,742.96
Interest as percentage of principal:
19.572%

Table 15–1–A

Payment Number	Principal	Interest	Cumulative Principal	Cumulative Interest	Principal Balance
1	$1,392.86	$600.00	$1,392.86	$600.00	$58,607.14
2	$1,406.79	$586.07	$2,799.65	$1,186.07	$57,200.35
3	$1,420.86	$572.00	$4,220.51	$1,758.07	$55,779.49
4	$1,435.07	$557.79	$5,655.58	$2,315.86	$54,344.42
5	$1,449.42	$543.44	$7,105.00	$2,859.30	$52,895.00
6	$1,463.91	$528.95	$8,568.91	$3,388.25	$51,431.09
7	$1,478.55	$514.31	$10,047.46	$3,902.56	$49,952.54
8	$1,493.33	$499.53	$11,540.79	$4,402.09	$48,459.21
9	$1,508.27	$484.59	$13,049.06	$4,886.68	$46,950.94
10	$1,523.35	$469.51	$14,572.41	$5,356.19	$45,427.59
11	$1,538.58	$454.28	$16,110.99	$5,810.47	$43,889.01
12	$1,553.97	$438.89	$17,664.96	$6,249.36	$42,335.04
13	$1,569.51	$423.35	$19,234.47	$6,672.71	$40,765.53
14	$1,585.20	$407.66	$20,819.67	$7,080.37	$39,180.33
15	$1,601.06	$391.80	$22,420.73	$7,472.17	$37,579.27
16	$1,617.07	$375.79	$24,037.80	$7,847.96	$35,962.20
17	$1,633.24	$359.62	$25,671.04	$8,207.58	$34,328.96
18	$1,649.57	$343.29	$27,320.61	$8,550.87	$32,679.39
19	$1,666.07	$326.79	$28,986.68	$8,877.66	$31,013.32
20	$1,682.73	$310.13	$30,669.41	$9,187.79	$29,330.59
21	$1,699.55	$293.31	$32,368.96	$9,481.10	$27,631.04
22	$1,716.55	$276.31	$34,085.51	$9,757.41	$25,914.49
23	$1,733.72	$259.14	$35,819.23	$10,016.55	$24,180.77
24	$1,751.05	$241.81	$37,570.28	$10,258.36	$22,429.72
25	$1,768.56	$224.30	$39,338.84	$10,482.66	$20,661.16
26	$1,786.25	$206.61	$41,125.09	$10,689.27	$18,874.91
27	$1,804.11	$188.75	$42,929.20	$10,878.02	$17,070.80
28	$1,822.15	$170.71	$44,751.35	$11,048.73	$15,248.65
29	$1,840.37	$152.49	$46,591.72	$11,201.22	$13,408.28
30	$1,858.78	$134.08	$48,450.50	$11,335.30	$11,549.50
31	$1,877.37	$115.49	$50,327.87	$11,450.79	$9,672.13
32	$1,896.14	$96.72	$52,224.01	$11,547.51	$7,775.99
33	$1,915.10	$77.76	$54,139.11	$11,625.27	$5,860.89
34	$1,934.25	$58.61	$56,073.36	$11,683.88	$3,926.64
35	$1,953.59	$39.27	$58,026.95	$11,723.15	$1,973.05
36	*$1,973.05	$19.73	$60,000.00	$11,742.88	$0.00

*The final payment has been adjusted to account for payments having been rounded to the nearest cent.

Owning Versus Leasing Equipment

PURCHASING EQUIPMENT

Purchasing equipment means taking title to, or assuming ownership of, the item. In this case, the asset representing the equipment is recorded on the organization's balance sheet. The purchase could take place by paying cash from the organization's cash reserves, or the organization could finance all or part of the purchase. If financing occurs, the resulting liability is also recorded on the balance sheet.

LEASING EQUIPMENT

When is a lease not a lease? When it is a lease-purchase, also known as a financial lease. This is a very real question that affects business decisions. The financial lease is described in the next section, and it is followed by a description of the operating lease.

Financial Lease

The lease-purchase is a formal agreement that may be called a lease, but it is really a contract to purchase. This contract-to-purchase transaction is also called a financial lease. The important difference is this: the equipment must be recorded on the books of the organization as a purchase. This process is called "capitalizing" the lease.

A financial lease is considered a contract to purchase. Generally speaking, a lease must be capitalized and thus placed on the balance sheet as an asset, with a corresponding liability, if the lease contract meets any one of the following criteria. These criteria include the following:

1. The lessee can buy the asset at the end of the lease term for a bargain price.

2. The lease transfers ownership to the lessee before the lease expires.
3. The lease lasts for 75 percent or more of the asset's estimated useful life.
4. The present value of the lease payments is 90 percent or more of the asset's value.

Operating Lease

The cost of an operating lease is considered an operating expense. It does not have to be capitalized and placed on the balance sheet because it does not meet the criteria just described.

An operating lease is treated as an expense of current operations. This is in contrast to the financial lease just described that is treated as an asset and a liability. A payment on an operating lease becomes an operating expense within the time period when the payment is made.

BUY-OR-LEASE MANAGEMENT DECISIONS

Leasing is an alternative to other means of financing. When analyzing lease-versus-purchase decisions, it is usually assumed that the money to purchase the equipment will be borrowed. In some cases, however, this is not true. The organization might decide to use cash from its own funds to make the purchase. This decision would, of course, change certain assumptions in the comparative analysis.

Another differential in comparative analysis concerns service agreements. Sometimes the service contracts or service agreements (to service and/or repair the equipment) are made a part of the lease agreement. This feature would need to be deleted from the total agreement before the comparison between leasing and purchasing can occur.

Why? Because the service agreement would be an expense, regardless of whether the equipment would be leased or purchased.

An Example

The question for our example is whether a clinic should purchase or lease equipment. We examine two clinics: Northside Clinic, a for-profit corporation, and Southside Clinic, a not-for-profit corporation.

For both Northside and Southside, assume that the equipment's cost will be $50,000 if it is purchased. Likewise, assume for both Northside and Southside that if the equipment is leased, the lease will amount to $11,000 per year for five years.

We also need to make assumptions about depreciation expense for the purchased equipment. We further assume straight-line depreciation in the amount of $10,000 for years 2 through 4. For the initial year of acquisition (year 0), we assume the half-year method of depreciation, whereby the amount will be one half of $10,000 or $5,000. We will further assume the purchased equipment will be sold for its salvage value of ten percent or $5,000 on the first day of year 5. (Therefore, the full amount of [prior] year 4's depreciation can be taken.)

The difference between the for-profit Northside and the not-for-profit Southside is that the for-profit is subject to income tax. We assume the federal and state income taxes will amount to a total of 25 percent. Thus, the depreciation taken as an expense results in a tax savings amounting to one quarter of the total expense in each year. The depreciation expense and its equivalent tax savings are shown by year in Table 16–1. Also, the same rationale is applicable for the leasing expense in the for-profit organization.

Table 16–1 Depreciation Expense Computation

	Year 0	Year 1	Year 2	Year 3	Year 4	Year 5
Depreciation expense	$5,000	$10,000	$10,000	$10,000	$10,000	—
Depreciation expense tax savings	$1,250	$2,500	$2,500	$2,500	$2,500	—

In the following section, we compare two financial situations that affect the way the analysis is performed: a for-profit, or proprietary, clinic and a not-for-profit clinic. For purposes of this analysis, what is the major difference? As we have previously stated, the for-profit practice realizes tax savings on expense items such as depreciation. The not-for-profit clinic does not realize such tax savings because it does not pay taxes. Consequently, one analysis later here (the for-profit) includes the effect of tax savings on depreciation, and the other analysis (the not-for-profit) has does not.

Computing the Comparative Net Cash Flow Effects of Owning Versus Leasing

This description results in computation of the net cash flow for owned equipment versus leased equipment in a for-profit organization compared with that of a not-for-profit organization. Tables 16–2–A.1 and 16–2–A.2 first illustrate the comparative net cash flow effects of owning versus leasing in a for-profit organization. Table 16–2–A.1 illustrates the cost of owning. The equipment purchase price of 50,000 in year 0 (line 1) and the salvage value of 5,000 in year 5 (line 3) are shown. The for-profit's net cash flow is also affected by tax savings from depreciation expense, as was previously explained and as is shown on line 2. The resulting net cash flow by year is shown on line 4.

Table 16–2–A.2 illustrates the cost of leasing in the for-profit organization. The equipment lease or rental payments are shown on line 5. The for-profit's net cash flow is affected by tax savings from the lease payments, as is shown on line 6. The resulting net cash flow by year is shown on line 7.

Tables 16–2–B.1 and 16–2–B.2 now illustrate the comparative net cash flow effects of owning versus leasing for the not-for-profit organization. Table 16–2–B.1 illustrates the cost of owning. The equipment purchase price of $50,000 in year 0 (line 8) and the salvage value of $5,000 in year 5 (line 10) are shown. The not-for-profit's net cash flow is not affected by tax savings from depreciation expense because it is exempt from such income taxes. Therefore, the depreciation expense tax savings entry on line 9 is shown as not applicable, or "n/a." The resulting net cash flow by year is then shown on line 11.

Table 16–2–B.2 illustrates the cost of leasing in the not-for-profit organization. The equipment lease or rental payments are shown on line 12. The not-for-profit's net cash flow is not affected by tax savings from the lease payments because it is exempt from such income taxes. Therefore, the lease expense tax savings entry on line 13 is shown as not applicable, or "n/a." The resulting net cash flow by year is then shown on line 14.

Table 16–2–A.1 Cost of Owning—Northside Clinic (For-Profit)—Comparative Cash Flow

Line Number		Year 0	Year 1	Year 2	Year 3	Year 4	Year 5
1	Equipment purchase price	($50,000)					
2	Depreciation expense tax savings	$1,250	$2,500	$2,500	$2,500	$2,500	—
3	Salvage value	—	—	—	—	—	$5,000
4	Net Cash Flow	($48,750)	$2,500	$2,500	$2,500	$2,500	$5,000

Table 16–2–A.2 Cost of Leasing—Northside Clinic (For-Profit)—Comparative Cash Flow

Line Number		Year 0	Year 1	Year 2	Year 3	Year 4	Year 5
5	Equipment lease (rental) payments	($11,000)	($11,000)	($11,000)	($11,000)	($11,000)	—
6	Lease expense tax savings	$2,750	$2,750	$2,750	$2,750	$2,750	—
7	Net Cash Flow	($8,250)	($8,250)	($8,250)	($8,250)	($8,250)	—

Table 16–2–B.1 Cost of Owning—Southside Clinic (Not-For-Profit)—Comparative Cash Flow

Line Number		Year 0	Year 1	Year 2	Year 3	Year 4	Year 5
8	Equipment purchase price	($50,000)					
9	Depreciation expense tax savings	n/a	n/a	n/a	n/a	n/a	—
10	Salvage value	—	—	—	—	—	$5,000
11	Net Cash Flow	($50,000)	—	—	—	—	$5,000

Table 16–2–B.2 Cost of Leasing—Southside Clinic (Not-For-Profit)—Comparative Cash Flow

Line Number		Year 0	Year 1	Year 2	Year 3	Year 4	Year 5
12	Equipment lease (rental) payments	($11,000)	($11,000)	($11,000)	($11,000)	($11,000)	—
13	Lease expense tax savings	n/a	n/a	n/a	n/a	n/a	—
14	Net Cash Flow	($11,000)	($11,000)	($11,000)	($11,000)	($11,000)	—

Computing the Comparative Present Value Cost of Owning Versus Cost of Leasing

This continuing description results in computation of the present value cost of owning versus leasing equipment in a for-profit organization compared with that of a not-for-profit organization.

Tables 16–2–C.1 and 16–2–C.2 now illustrate the present value cost of owning versus leasing for the for-profit organization. Table 16–2–C.1 first carries forward (on line 15) the net cash flow computed on line 4. Line 16 then shows the present value factor for each year at 8 percent, which is the assumed cost of capital in this example. Line 17 contains the present value answers, which result

from multiplying line 15 times line 16. The overall present value cost of owning (derived by adding all items on line 17) is shown on line 18.

Table 16–2–C.2 illustrates the present value cost of leasing in the for-profit organization. Table 16–2–C.2 first carries forward (on line 19) the net cash flow computed on line 7. Line 20 then shows the present value factor for each year at 8 percent, which is the assumed cost of capital in this example. Line 21 contains the present value answers, which result from multiplying line 19 times line 20. The overall present value cost of owning (derived by adding all items on line 21) is shown on line 22.

Finally, Table 16–2–C.3 compares the for-profit organization's cost of owning to its

Table 16–2–C.1 Cost of Owning—Northside Clinic (For-Profit)—Comparative Present Value

Line Number	For-Profit Cost of Owning	Year 0	Year 1	Year 2	Year 3	Year 4	Year 5
15	Net Cash Flow (from line 4)	($48,750)	$2,500	$2,500	$2,500	$2,500	$5,000
16	Present value factor (at 8%)	n/a	0.926	0.857	0.794	0.735	0.681
17	Present value answers =	($48,750)	$2,315	$2,143	$1,985	$1,838	$3,405
18	Present value cost of owning =	($37,064)					

Table 16–2–C.2 Cost of Leasing—Northside Clinic (For-Profit)—Comparative Present Value

Line Number	For-Profit Cost of Leasing	Year 0	Year 1	Year 2	Year 3	Year 4	Year 5
19	Net cash flow (from line 7)	($8,250)	($8,250)	($8,250)	($8,250)	($8,250)	—
20	Present value factor (at 8%)	n/a	0.926	0.857	0.794	0.735	—
21	Present value answers =	($8,250)	($7,640)	($7,070)	($6,551)	($6,064)	—
22	Present value cost of leasing =	($35,575)					

Table 16–2–C.3 Comparison of Costs-Northside Clinic (For-Profit)

Line Number	Computation of Difference
23 Net advantage to leasing = $1,489	(37,064)(line 18) less (35,575)(line 22) equals 1,489

cost of leasing. In the case of the for-profit, the net advantage is to leasing by a net amount of $1,489. The tables now illustrate the present value cost of owning versus leasing for the not-for-profit organization. Table 16–2–D.1 illustrates the present value cost of owning. It first carries forward (on line 24) the net cash flow computed on line 11. Line 25 then shows the present value factor for each year at 8 percent, which is the assumed cost of capital in this example. Line 26 contains the present value answers, which result from multiplying line 24 times line 25. The overall present value cost of owning (derived by adding all items on line 26) is shown on line 27.

Table 16–2–D.2 illustrates the present value cost of leasing in the not-for-profit organization. It first carries forward (on line 28) the net cash flow computed on line 14. Line 29 then shows the present value factor for each year at 8 percent, which is the assumed cost of capital in this example. Line 30 contains the present value answers, which result from multiplying line 28 times line 29. The overall present value cost of owning, (derived by adding all items on line 30) is shown on line 31.

Finally, Table 16–2–D.3 compares the not-for-profit organization's cost of owning to its cost of leasing. In the case of the not-for-profit, the net advantage is to owning by

---

Table 16–2–D.1 Cost of Owning—Southside Clinic (Not-For-Profit)—Comparative Present Value

Line Number	Not-For-Profit Cost of Owning	Year 0	Year 1	Year 2	Year 3	Year 4	Year 5
24	Net cash flow (from line 11)	($50,000)	—	—	—	—	$5,000
25	Present value factor (at 8%)	n/a	—	—	—	—	0.681
26	Present value answer =	($50,000)	—	—	—	—	$3,405
27	Present value cost of owning =	($46,595)					

Table 16–2–D.1 Cost of Leasing—Southside Clinic (Not-For-Profit)—Comparative Present Value

Line Number	Not-For-Profit Cost of Leasing	Year 0	Year 1	Year 2	Year 3	Year 4	Year 5
28	Net cash flow (from line 14)	($11,000)	($11,000)	($11,000)	($11,000)	($11,000)	—
29	Present value factor (at 8%)	n/a	0.926	0.857	0.794	0.735	
30	Present value answer =	($11,000)	($10,186)	($9,427)	($8,573)	($8,085)	—
31	Present value cost of leasing =	($47,271)					

Table 16–2–D.3 Comparison of Costs—Southside Clinic (Not-For-Profit)

Line Number	Computation of Difference
32 Net Advantage to Owning = 676	(47,271)(line 31) less (46,595)(line 27) equals 676

a net amount of $676. It might be noted that the net difference of $676 is so small that it might be disregarded and considered as a nearly neutral comparison between the two methods of financing.

In summary, the tax effect on cash flow of for-profit versus not-for-profit will generally (but not always) be taken into account in comparative proposals for funding.

 INFORMATION CHECKPOINT

What Is Needed?	An example of a buy-or-lease management decision analysis.
Where Is It Found?	Probably with your manager or your departmental director.
How Is It Used?	Study the way the analysis is laid out and the method of comparison used.

 KEY TERMS

Buy-or-Lease Decisions
Depreciation
Equipment Purchase
Financial Lease
For-Profit Organization
Lease-Purchase
Not-for-Profit Organization
Operating Lease
Present Value

 DISCUSSION QUESTIONS

1. In the examples given in the chapter, there is not much monetary difference between owning versus leasing. In these circumstances, which method would you recommend? Why?
2. Have you ever been involved in a lease-or-buy decision in business? In your personal life?
3. If so, was the decision made in a formal reporting format, or as an informal decision?
4. Do you think this was the best way to make the decision? If not, what would you change? Why?

CHAPTER 17

Putting It All Together: Creating a Business Plan

PROGRESS NOTES

After completing this chapter you should be able to

1. Understand the construction of a business plan.
2. Describe the organization segment of a business plan.
3. Describe the marketing segment of a business plan.
4. Describe the financial segment of a business plan.

OVERVIEW

A business plan is a document, typically prepared in order to obtain funding and/or financing. A traditional business plan typically contains information about three major elements: the proposed project's organization, marketing, and financial aspects. However, the actual business plan is generally constructed in a series of segments, each involving a particular type of information. The overall business plan is built up as these individual segments are completed. The segments are described in this chapter.

ELEMENTS OF THE BUSINESS PLAN

A traditional business plan typically contains three major elements:

- Organization plan
- Marketing plan
- Financial plan

The organization segment should describe the management team. The marketing segment should discuss who may use the service and/or product. The financial segment should contain the numbers that illustrate how the project is expected to operate over an initial period of time. We believe that it is also important to begin the business plan with an executive summary that outlines key points, plus a clear and concise description of the service and/or product that is the subject of the plan.

PREPARING TO CONSTRUCT THE BUSINESS PLAN

The planning stage will shape a business plan's content. The initial decisions, such as those shown in Exhibit 17–1, will determine your approach to the plan. For example, if your organization requires a certain type of format and pre-existing blank spreadsheets, many of the initial decisions have already

163

Exhibit 17–1 Initial Decisions for the Business Plan

Business Plan Initial Decisions

- Outline necessary format
- Decide on length
- Decide on level of sophistication
- Determine what information is needed
- Determine who will provide each piece of information

Courtesy of Baker and Baker, Dallas, Texas

been made for you. Otherwise, the checklist contained in Exhibit 17–1 will assist you in making initial decisions for the business plan's approach.

It is important to note that the level of sophistication for the overall plan should be based on the decision makers who will be the primary audience. Another practical consideration involves creating a grid or matrix to assist in gathering all necessary information. The grid or matrix could also include which individuals are responsible for helping to create or collect the required information. Finally, it is important to create a file at the beginning of the project in which all computations, backup information, dates, and sources are kept together in an organized fashion.

THE SERVICE OR EQUIPMENT DESCRIPTION

The service and/or equipment description should do a good job of describing what the heart of the business plan is about. If the business plan is for a project or a new service line, then this description would expand to include the entire project or the overall service line. Information that should always be included in the description is contained in Exhibit 17–2.

The test of a good description is whether an individual who has never been involved in your planning can read the description and understand it without additional questions being raised.

THE ORGANIZATION SEGMENT

The organization segment should describe the management team. But it should also describe how the proposed service or equipment fits into the organization. Who will be charged with the new budget? Who will be responsible for the controls and reporting for this proposal? It is important to provide a clear picture that informs decision makers about how the proposed acquisition will be managed. Basic facts to explain are included in Exhibit 17–3.

Exhibit 17–2 Basic Information for the Service or Equipment Description

Service or Equipment Description

- What the service specifically provides
- Why this service is different and /or special
- What the equipment specifically does
- Why this equipment is different and/or special
- Required training, if applicable
- Regulatory requirements and/or impact, if any

Courtesy of Baker and Baker, Dallas, Texas

Exhibit 17–3 Basic Information for the Organization Segment

Organization Segment Information

- Physical location where service will be provided
- Physical location of the equipment
- The department responsible for the budget
- The division responsible for operations
- The directly responsible supervisor
- Composition of the overall management team

  Courtesy of Baker and Baker, Dallas, Texas

Exhibit 17–4 Basic Information for the Marketing Segment

Marketing Segment Information

- Physicians who will use the service or equipment

- New patients who will use the service or equipment

- Established patients who will use the service or equipment

- Estimated portion of the market to be captured

- Competition and its impact

  Courtesy of Baker and Baker, Dallas, Texas

Visual depictions of the chain of authority and supervisory responsibilities provide helpful illustrations for this segment.

THE MARKETING SEGMENT

The marketing segment should describe the available market, that portion of the market your service or equipment should attract, and that portion of the market occupied by the competition. This segment should achieve a balance between describing those individuals who will be availing themselves of the service or equipment and a description of the competition. A description of who will be responsible for the marketing is also valuable information for the decision makers. Strive for a realistic and objective appraisal of the situation. Basic facts to include are illustrated in Exhibit 17–4.

Of all areas of the business plan, the marketing segment is most likely to be overoptimistic in its assumptions. It is wise to be conservative about estimations of physician

and patient acceptance and usage. And it is equally wise to be realistic when assessing the competition and its likely impact.

THE FINANCIAL ANALYSIS SEGMENT

The financial segment should contain the numbers that illustrate how the project is expected to operate over an initial period of time. Financial plans may range from a projected period of one year to as much as ten years. A one-year projection is often too short to show true outcomes, whereas a ten-year projection may be too long to meaningfully forecast. Your organization will usually have a standard length of time that is accepted for these projections. The standard forecasted periods for high-tech equipment, for example, often range from three to five years. Why? Because advances in technology may render them obsolete in five years or less. Therefore, the forecast is set for a realistically short time period.

The financial analysis for a business plan should contain a forecast of operations. The forecast may be simple, such as a cash flow statement, or it may be more extensive. A more extensive forecast would also require a balance sheet and an income statement. The required statements and schedules will depend on two factors: the size and complexity of the project and the usual procedure for a business plan presentation that is expected in your organization.

The Projected Cash Flow Statement

As we have just stated, it is possible that the forecast of operations may simply consist of the cash flow statement. In any case, the statement can be complex, with many detailed line items, or it can be condensed. The condensed type of statement is most often found in a business plan. Keep in mind, however, that a detailed worksheet—the source of the information on the condensed statement—may well be filed in the supporting work papers for the project. Necessary cash flow assumptions are illustrated in Exhibit 17–5.

Exhibit 17–5 Basic Assumptions for the Cash Flow Statement

Cash Flow Statement Assumptions
• Number of years in the future to forecast • Capital asset purchase or lease information • Capital asset salvage value (if any) • Cash inflow • Cash outflow • Cost of capital (if applicable)
Courtesy of Baker and Baker, Dallas, Texas

The Projected Income Statement

What income statement assumptions will your business plan's financial analysis require? The basic assumptions for a health care project's income statement are illustrated in Exhibit 17–6.

The "revenue type" in Exhibit 17–6 refers to whether, for example, the revenue is derived entirely from services or whether part of the revenue is derived from drugs and devices. The "revenue sources" refers to how many payers will pay for the service and/or drug and device and in what proportion (such as Medicare 60 percent, Medicaid 15 percent, and commercial payers 25 percent). The "revenue amount" refers to how much each payer is expected to pay for the service and/or drug and device. The total amount of revenue can then be determined by multiplying each payer's expected payment rate times the percentage of the total represented by that payer.

In regard to the "expenses" in Exhibit 17–6, the labor cost will usually be deter-

Exhibit 17–6 Basic Assumptions for the Income Statement

Income Statement Assumptions
• Revenue type • Revenue source(s) • Revenue amount • Expenses: • Labor • Supplies • Cost of drug or device (if applicable) • Equipment • Space occupancy • Overhead
Courtesy of Baker and Baker, Dallas, Texas

mined by staffing assumptions. The required staffing should be set out by type of employee and the pay rate for each type of employee. The number of full-time equivalents for each type of employee will then be established. The FTEs will be multiplied times the assumed pay rate to arrive at the labor cost assumption.

"Supplies" refers to the necessary supplies required to perform the procedure or service. "Cost of drug or device" refers to the cost to the organization of purchasing the drug or device (if a drug or device is necessary to the service). The labor, supplies, and cost of drug or device are costs that can be directly attributed to the service that is that subject of the business plan. Likewise, the "equipment" cost refers to the annual depreciation expense of any equipment that is directly attributed to the service that is the subject of the business plan.

"Space occupancy" refers to the overall cost of occupying the space required for the service or procedure. "Space occupancy" is a catchall phrase. It includes either annual depreciation expense (if the building is owned) or annual rent expense (if the building is leased) of the square footage required for the service. Space occupancy also includes other related costs such as utilities, maintenance, housekeeping, and insurance. Security might also be included in this category. The actual forecast might group these expense items into one line item, or the forecast might show each individual expense (depreciation, housekeeping, etc.) on a separate line. If the expenses are grouped, a footnote or a supplemental schedule should show the actual detail that makes up the total amount.

"Overhead" refers to the remaining expenses of operation that are necessary to produce the service but that are not directly attributable to that service. Examples of such overhead in a physician's office might include items such as postage and copy paper. This amount of indirect overhead may be expressed as a percentage; for example, "overhead equals ten percent." Whether the "space occupancy" example or the "overhead" example discussed previously here are grouped or detailed in the forecast will probably depend on how large the amount is in relation to the other expenses, or it might depend instead on the usual format that your organization expects to see in a typical business plan that is presented to management.

The Projected Balance Sheet

What balance sheet assumptions will your business plan's financial analysis require? The basic assumptions for a health care project's balance sheet are illustrated in Exhibit 17–7.

The elements of a balance sheet (assets, liabilities, and equity) are described in a previous chapter. If a full projected set of statements is required for the business plan, the

---

Exhibit 17–7 Basic Assumptions for the Balance Sheet

Balance Sheet Assumptions

- Cash
- Accounts Receivable
- Inventories
- Property and Equipment
- Accounts Payable
- Accrued Current Liabilities
- Long-Term Liabilities
- Equity

Courtesy of Baker and Baker, Dallas, Texas

balance sheet entries will in large part be a function of the income statement projections discussed in the preceding section of this chapter. For example, accounts receivable would be primarily determined by the revenue assumptions, while accounts payable would be primarily determined by the expense assumptions. Likewise, acquisition of equipment or other capital assets will affect capital assets (property and equipment), while their funding assumptions will affect either or both liability and equity totals on the projected balance sheet.

THE "KNOWLEDGEABLE READER" APPROACH TO YOUR BUSINESS PLAN

We believe a good business plan should answer the questions that occur to a knowledgeable reader. Thus, the information you include in the business plan should reflect the choices that you made in selecting the assumptions for your financial analysis. For instance, an example of considerations for forecasting an equipment acquisition is presented in Exhibit 17–8. The final business plan content should touch upon these points in describing your assumptions that underlie the financial analysis.

THE EXECUTIVE SUMMARY

The executive summary should contain a well-written and concise summary of the entire plan. It should not be longer than two pages; many decision makers consider one page desirable. Some people like to write the executive summary first. They tend to use it as an outline to guide the rest of the content. Other people like to write the executive summary last, when they know what all the detailed content contains. In either

Exhibit 17–8 Considerations for Forecasting Equipment Acquisition

Considerations for Forecasting Equipment Acquisition

- Only one location?
- Equipment single purpose or multipurpose?
- Technology: new, middle-aged, old (obsolete vs. untested)?
- Equipment compatibility?
- Medical supply cost?
- High or low capital investment?
- Buy new or used (refurbished)?
- Buy or lease?
- Lease for number of years or lease on a pay-per-procedure deal?
- How much staff training is required?
- Certification required?
- Square footage required for equipment?
- Is the required square footage available?
- Cleaning methods and equipment (and staff level required)?
- Repairs and maintenance expense (high, medium, low)?

Courtesy of Baker and Baker, Dallas, Texas

instance, the executive summary should tell the entire story in a compelling manner.

ASSEMBLING THE BUSINESS PLAN

The business plan should be assembled into a suitable report format that is determined by many of your initial decisions, such as length and level of sophistication. A sample format appears in Exhibit 17–9.

If an appendix is desired, it should contain detail to support certain contents in the main part of the business plan. In preparing

Exhibit 17–9 Sample Format for a Business Plan

A Sample Business Plan Format

- Title Page
- Table of Contents
- Executive Summary
- Service and/or Equipment Description
- The Organizational Plan
- The Marketing Plan
- The Financial Plan
- Appendix (optional)

Courtesy of Baker and Baker, Dallas, Texas

the final report, certain other logistics are important. It is expected, for example, that the pages should be numbered. (You might also want to add the date in the footer and perhaps a version number as well.) Although the report may or may not be bound, it should have all pages firmly secured.

PRESENTING THE BUSINESS PLAN

You may be asked to present more than once. Sometimes you will have to prepare a short form and a long form of the plan, depending on the audience. Tips on presenting your business plan are presented in Exhibit 17–10.

It is especially important to practice your presentation in advance. When you leave time for questions and for discussion, you also want to be well prepared for anticipated questions. By constructing a well-thought-out business plan, you have substantially increased your chances for a successful outcome.

Exhibit 17–10 Tips on Presentation of the Business Plan

Tips on Presenting Your Business Plan

- Determine who will be attending ahead of time
- Determine how long you will have for the presentation
- Be sure you have a copy for each attendee
- Decide upon whether to use audio visual aids
  - LCD projector and PowerPoint slides?
  - Flip chart and markers?
  - Other methods?
- Practice your presentation in advance
- Leave time for questions and for discussion

Courtesy of Baker and Baker, Dallas, Texas

 INFORMATION CHECKPOINT

What Is Needed?	A sample of a business plan.
Where Is It Found?	Probably with your manager or the departmental director.
How Is It Used?	Study the way the business plan was distributed. Who received it? What did they do with it? What was the result?

KEY TERMS

Business Plan
Overhead
Revenue Amount
Revenue Sources
Revenue Type
Space Occupancy
Supplies

 DISCUSSION QUESTIONS

1. Have you ever been involved in the creation of a business plan?
2. If so, did the plan include all three segments (organizational, marketing, and finance)? If not, why do you think one or more of the segments was missing?
3. Have you ever attended the formal presentation of a business plan? If so, was it successful in obtaining the desired funding?
4. Was the plan that was presented similar to what we have described in this chapter? What would you have changed in the presentation? Why?

PART VII

Case Study

CHAPTER 18

Case Study:
Metropolis Health System

BACKGROUND

1. The Hospital System

Metropolis Health System (MHS) offers comprehensive health care services. It is a midsize taxing district hospital. Although MHS has the power to raise revenues through taxes, it has not done so for the past seven years.

2. The Area

MHS is located in the town of Metropolis, which has a population of 50,000. The town has a small college and a modest number of environmentally clean industries.

3. MHS Services

MHS has taken significant steps to reduce hospital stays. It has developed a comprehensive array of services that are accessible, cost-effective, and responsive to the community's needs. These services are wellness oriented in that they strive for prevention rather than treatment. As a result of these steps, inpatient visits have increased overall by only 1,000 per year since 1998, whereas outpatient/same-day sur-

gery visits have had an increase of over 50,000 per year.

A number of programmatic, service, and facility enhancements support this major transition in the community's institutional health care. They are geared to provide the quality, convenience, affordability, and personal care that best suit the health needs of the people whom MHS serves.

- *Rehabilitation and Wellness Center*—for outpatient physical therapy and return-to-work services plus cardiac and pulmonary rehabilitation to get people back to a normal way of living.
- *Home Health Services*—bringing skilled care, therapy, and medical social services into the home; a comfortable and affordable alternative in longer term care.
- *Same-Day Surgery (SDS)*—eliminating the need for an overnight stay. Since 1998, same-day surgery procedures have doubled at MHS.
- *Skilled Nursing Facility*—inpatient service to assist patients in returning more fully to an independent lifestyle.
- *Community Health and Wellness*—community health outreach programs that

provide educational seminars on a variety of health issues, a diabetes education center, support services for patients with cancer, health awareness events, and a women's health resource center.

- *Occupational Health Services*—helping to reduce workplace injury costs at over 100 area businesses through consultation on injury avoidance and work-specific rehabilitation services.
- *Recovery Services*—offering mental health services, including substance abuse programs and support groups along with individual and family counseling.

4. MHS's Plant

The central building for the hospital is in the center of a two–square block area. A physicians' office building is to the west. Two administrative offices, converted from former residences, are on one corner. The new ambulatory center, completed two years ago, has an *L* shape and sits on one corner of the western block. A laundry and maintenance building sits on the extreme back of the property. A four-story parking garage is located on the eastern back corner. An employee parking lot sits beside the laundry and maintenance building. Visitor parking lots fill the front eastern portion of the property. A helipad is on the extreme western edge of the property behind the physicians' office building.

5. MHS Board of Trustee

Eight local community leaders who bring diverse skills to the board govern MHS. The trustees generously volunteer their time to plan the strategic direction of MHS, thus ensuring the system's ability to provide quality comprehensive health care to the community.

6. MHS Management

A chief executive officer manages MHS. Seven senior vice presidents report to the CEO. MHS is organized into 23 major responsibility centers.

7. MHS Employees

All 500 team members employed by MHS are integral to achieving the high standards for which the system strives. The quality improvement program, implemented in 1995, is aimed at meeting client needs sooner, better, and more cost-effectively. Participants in the program are from all areas of the system.

8. MHS Physicians

The MHS medical staff is a key part of MHS's ability to provide excellence in health care. Over 75 physicians cover more than 30 medical specialties. The high quality of their training and their commitment to the practice of medicine are great assets to the health of the community.

The physicians are very much a part of MHS's drive for continual improvement on the quality health care services offered in the community. MHS brings in medical experts from around the country to provide training in new techniques, made possible by MHS's technologic advancements. MHS also ensures that physicians are offered seminars, symposiums, and continuing education programs that permit them to remain current with changes in the medical field.

The medical staff's quality improvement program has begun a care path initiative to track effective means for diagnosis, treatment, and follow-up. This initiative will help avoid unnecessary or duplicate use of expensive medications or technologies.

9. MHS Foundation

Metropolis Health Foundation is presently being created to serve as the philanthropic arm of MHS. It will operate in a separate corporation governed by a board of 12 community leaders and supported by a 15-member special events board. The mission of the foundation will be to secure financial and nonfinancial support for realizing the MHS vision of providing comprehensive health care for the community.

Funds donated by individuals, businesses, foundations, and organizations will be designated for a variety of purposes at MHS, including the operations of specific departments, community outreach programs, continuing education for employees, endowment, equipment, and capital improvements.

10. MHS Volunteer Auxiliary

There are 500 volunteers who provide over 60,000 hours of service to MHS each year. These men and women assist in virtually every part of the system's operations. They also conduct community programs on behalf of MHS.

The auxiliary funds its programs and makes financial contributions to MHS through money it raises on renting televisions and vending gifts and other items at the hospital. In the past, its donations to MHS have generally been designated for medical equipment purchases. The auxiliary has given $250,000 over the last five years.

11. Planning the Future for MHS

The MHS has identified five areas of desired service and programmatic enhancement in its five-year strategic plan:

   I. Ambulatory Services
  II. Physical Medicine and Rehabilitative Services
 III. Cardiovascular Services
 IV. Oncology Services
  V. Community Health Services

MHS has set out to answer the most critical health needs that are specific to its community. Over the next five years, the MHS strategic plan will continue a tradition of quality, community-oriented health care to meet future demands.

12. Financing the Future

MHS has established a corporate depreciation fund. The fund's purpose is to ease the financial burden of replacing fixed assets. Presently, it has almost $2 million for needed equipment or renovations.

I. MHS CASE STUDY

Financial Statements

- Balance Sheet (Exhibit 18–1)
- Statement of Revenue and Expense (Exhibit 18–2)
- Statement of Cash Flows (Exhibit 18–3)
- Statement of Changes in Fund Balance (Exhibit 18–4)
- Schedule of Property, Plant, and Equipment (Exhibit 18–5)
- Schedule of Patient Revenue (Exhibit 18–6)
- Schedule of Operating Expenses (Exhibit 18–7)

Statistics and Organizational Structure

- Statistics (Exhibit 18–8)
- MHS Nursing Practice and Administration Organization Chart (Figure 18–1)
- MHS Executive-Level Organization Chart (Figure 18–2)

Variance Analysis Report and Recommendations

- Radiology Diagnostic Clinic Report

Exhibit 18–1 Balance Sheet

<table>
<tr><td colspan="4" align="center">Metropolis Health System
Balance Sheet
March 31, 20X7</td></tr>
<tr><td>Assets</td><td></td><td>Liabilities and Fund Balance</td><td></td></tr>
<tr><td>Current Assets</td><td></td><td>Current Liabilities</td><td></td></tr>
<tr><td>Cash and Cash Equivalents</td><td>$1,150,000</td><td>Current Maturities of Long-Term</td><td></td></tr>
<tr><td>Assets Whose Use Is Limited</td><td>825,000</td><td> Debt</td><td>525,000</td></tr>
<tr><td>Patient Accounts Receivable</td><td>7,400,000</td><td>Accounts Payable and Accrued</td><td></td></tr>
<tr><td>(Net of $1,300,000 Allowance</td><td></td><td> Expenses</td><td>$4,900,000</td></tr>
<tr><td> for Bad Debts)</td><td></td><td>Bond Interest Payable</td><td>300,000</td></tr>
<tr><td>Other Receivables</td><td>150,000</td><td>Reimbursement Settlement</td><td></td></tr>
<tr><td></td><td></td><td> Payable</td><td>100,000</td></tr>
<tr><td>Inventories</td><td>900,000</td><td></td><td></td></tr>
<tr><td>Prepaid Expenses</td><td>200,000</td><td>Total Current Liabilities</td><td>5,825,000</td></tr>
<tr><td>Total Current Assets</td><td>10,625,000</td><td>Long-Term Debt</td><td>6,000,000</td></tr>
<tr><td></td><td></td><td>Less Current Portion of</td><td></td></tr>
<tr><td>Assets Whose Use Is Limited</td><td></td><td> Long-Term Debt</td><td><525,000></td></tr>
<tr><td>Corporate Funded</td><td></td><td>Net Long-Term Debt</td><td>5,475,000</td></tr>
<tr><td> Depreciation</td><td>1,950,000</td><td>Total Liabilities</td><td>11,300,000</td></tr>
<tr><td>Held by Trustee Under Bond</td><td></td><td></td><td></td></tr>
<tr><td> Indenture Agreement</td><td>1,425,000</td><td>Fund Balances</td><td></td></tr>
<tr><td></td><td></td><td>General Fund</td><td>21,500,000</td></tr>
<tr><td>Total Assets Whose Use Is</td><td></td><td></td><td></td></tr>
<tr><td> Limited</td><td>3,375,000</td><td>Total Fund Balances</td><td>21,500,000</td></tr>
<tr><td>Less Current Portion</td><td><825,000></td><td>Total Liabilities and Fund</td><td></td></tr>
<tr><td>Net Assets Whose Use Is</td><td></td><td> Balances</td><td>32,800,000</td></tr>
<tr><td> Limited</td><td>2,550,000</td><td></td><td></td></tr>
<tr><td>Property, Plant, and</td><td></td><td></td><td></td></tr>
<tr><td> Equipment, net</td><td>19,300,000</td><td></td><td></td></tr>
<tr><td>Other Assets</td><td>325,000</td><td></td><td></td></tr>
<tr><td>Total Assets</td><td>$32,800,000</td><td></td><td></td></tr>
</table>

Exhibit 18–2 Statement of Revenue and Expense

Metropolis Health System
Statement of Revenue and Expense
For the Year Ended March 31, 20X7

Revenue		
Net patient service revenue	$34,000,000	
Other revenue	1,100,000	
Total Operating Revenue		$35,100,000
Expenses		
Nursing services	$5,025,000	
Other professional services	13,100,000	
General services	3,200,000	
Support services	8,300,000	
Depreciation	1,900,000	
Amortization	50,000	
Interest	325,000	
Provision for doubtful accounts	1,500,000	
Total Expenses		33,400,000
Income from Operations		$1,700,000
Nonoperating Gains (Losses)		
Unrestricted gifts and memorials	$20,000	
Interest income	80,000	
Nonoperating Gains, Net		100,000
Revenue and Gains in Excess of Expenses and Losses		$1,800,000

Exhibit 18–3 Statement of Cash Flows

Metropolis Health System
Statement of Cash Flows
For the Year Ended March 31, 20X7

Statement of Cash Flows

Operating Activities	
Income from operations	$1,700,000
Adjustments to reconcile income from operations	
to net cash flows from operating activities	
Depreciation and amortization	1,950,000
Changes in asset and liability accounts	
Patient accounts receivable	250,000
Other receivables	<50,000>
Inventories	<50,000>
Prepaid expenses and other assets	<50,000>
Accounts payable and accrued expenses	<400,000>
Reduction of bond interest payable	<25,000>
Estimated third-party payer settlements	<75,000>
Interest income received	80,000
Unrestricted gifts and memorials received	20,000
Net cash flow from operating activities	$3,350,000
Cash Flows from Capital and Related Financing Activities	
Repayment of long-term obligations	<500,000>
Cash Flows from Investing Activities	
Purchase of assets whose use is limited	<100,000>
Equipment purchases and building improvements	<2,000,000>
Net Increase (Decrease) in Cash and Cash Equivalents	$750,000
Cash and Cash Equivalents, Beginning of Year	400,000
Cash and Cash Equivalents, End of Year	$1,150,000

Exhibit 18–4 Statement of Changes in Fund Balance

Metropolis Health System Statement of Changes in Fund Balance For the Year Ended March 31, 20X7	
General Fund Balance April 1, 1999	$19,700,000
Revenue and Gains in Excess of Expenses and Losses	1,800,000
General Fund Balance March 31, 2000	$21,500,000

Exhibit 18–5 Schedule of Property, Plant, and Equipment

Metropolis Health System Schedule of Property, Plant, and Equipment For the Year Ended March 31, 20X7	
Buildings and Improvements	$14,700,000
Land Improvements	1,100,000
Equipment	28,900,000
Total	$44,700,000
Less Accumulated Depreciation	(26,100,000)
Net Depreciable Assets	$18,600,000
Land	480,000
Construction in Progress	220,000
Net Property, Plant, and Equipment	$19,300,000

Exhibit 18–6 Schedule of Patient Revenue

Metropolis Health System
Schedule of Patient Revenue
For the Year Ended March 31, 20X7

Patient Services Revenue	
Routine revenue	$9,850,000
Laboratory	7,375,000
Radiology and CT scanner	5,825,000
OB–nursery	450,000
Pharmacy	3,175,000
Emergency service	2,200,000
Medical and surgical supply and IV	5,050,000
Operating rooms	5,250,000
Anesthesiology	1,600,000
Respiratory therapy	900,000
Physical therapy	1,475,000
EKG and EEG	1,050,000
Ambulance service	900,000
Oxygen	575,000
Home health and hospice	1,675,000
Substance abuse	375,000
Other	775,000
Subtotal	$48,500,000
Less allowances and charity care	14,500,000
Net Patient Service Revenue	$34,000,000

Exhibit 18–7 Schedule of Operating Expenses

Metropolis Health System
Schedule of Operating Expenses
For the Year Ended March 31, 20X7

Nursing Services		General Services	
Routine Medical-Surgical	$3,880,000	Dietary	$1,055,000
Operating Room	300,000	Maintenance	1,000,000
Intensive Care Units	395,000	Laundry	295,000
OB-Nursery	150,000	Housekeeping	470,000
Other	300,000	Security	50,000
Total	$5,025,000	Medical Records	330,000
		Total	$3,200,000
Other Professional Services			
Laboratory	$2,375,000	Support Services	
Radiology and CT Scanner	1,700,000	General	$4,600,000
Pharmacy	1,375,000	Insurance	240,000
Emergency Service	950,000	Payroll Taxes	1,130,000
Medical and Surgical Supply	1,800,000	Employee Welfare	1,900,000
Operating Rooms and		Other	430,000
Anesthesia	1,525,000	Total	$8,300,000
Respiratory Therapy	525,000		
Physical Therapy	700,000	Depreciation	1,900,000
EKG and EEG	185,000	Amortization	50,000
Ambulance Service	80,000		
Substance Abuse	460,000	Interest Expense	325,000
Home Health and Hospice	1,295,000		
Other	130,000	Provision for Doubtful	
Total	$13,100,000	Accounts	1,500,000
		Total Operating Expenses	$33,400,000

Exhibit 18–8 Hospital Statistical Data

Metropolis Health System
Schedule of Hospital Statistics
For the Year Ended March 31, 20X7

Inpatient Indicators:		Departmental Volume Indicators:	
Patient Days			
Medical and surgical	13650	Respiratory therapy treatments	51,480
Obstetrics	1080	Physical therapy treatments	34,050
Skilled nursing unit	4500	Laboratory workload units	
		(in thousands)	2,750
Admissions		EKGs	8,900
Adult acute care	3610	CT scans	2,780
Newborn	315	MRI scans	910
Skilled nursing unit	440	Emergency room visits	11,820
		Ambulance trips	2,320
Discharges		Home Health visits	14,950
Adult acute care	3580		
Newborn	315	Approximate number of employees	
Skilled nursing unit	445	(FTE)	510
Average Length of Stay (in days)	4.1		

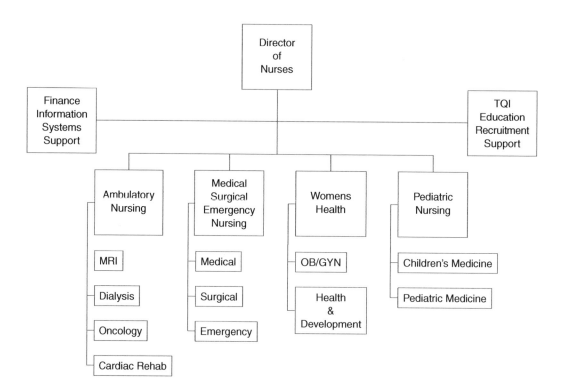

Figure 18–1 MHS Nursing Practice and Administration Organization Chart. Courtesy of Resource Group, Ltd., Dallas, Texas.

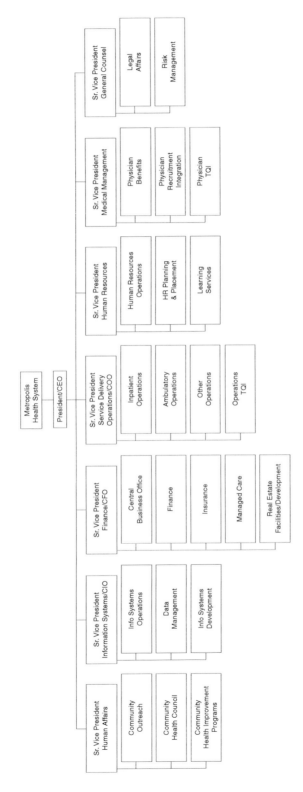

Figure 18–2 MHS Executive-Level Organization Chart. Courtesy of Resource Group, Ltd., Dallas, Texas.

Using Financial Ratios and Benchmarking: A Case Study in Comparative Analysis

Sample Hospital is another facility within the Metropolis Health System. Sample Hospital has recently been acquired by Metropolis. It is a 100-bed hospital that has been losing money steadily over the last several years. The new chief financial officer (CFO) has decided to use benchmarking as an aid to turn around Sample's financial situation. Benchmarking will illustrate where the hospital stands in relationship to its peer group.

The CFO orders two benchmarking reports: one for the hospitals that are 100 beds or less and one for all hospitals, no matter the size. The 100 beds or less report will allow direct comparability for Sample, while the all-hospital report will give a universal or overall view of Sample's standing. Both reports appear at the end of this case study. Exhibit 18–A–1 is the benchmark data report for Sample General Hospital compared with hospitals less than 100 beds, whereas Exhibit 18–A–2 is the benchmark data report for Sample General Hospital compared with all hospitals.

When the reports arrive, the CFO writes a description of how the data are arranged so that his managers will better understand the information presented. His description includes the following points:

1. The percentile rankings are intended to present the hospital's performance ranked against all other performers in the comparison group. Whether the hospital's actual performance is good or bad depends on the statistic being evaluated.

2. The first column, labeled "Year 1," provides a historical trend of actual performance of the hospital in the previous year. It is provided for reference only so that the reader can see the trend over time.

3. The column labeled "Q1 Year 2" represents the first quarter of the current year. These are the most recent data that this service has been provided for Sample Hospital and are the data used in the comparison columns that follow.

4. The column labeled "Benchmark: 50th Percentile" represents the 50th percentile of all of the hospitals in the comparison group that supplied data for the individual line item.

5. The "Variance" column compares the data from Q1 Year 2 of Sample Hospital with the 50th percentile information from the entire comparison group.

6. The column labeled "Range" indicates where Sample Hospital's individual score fell within a percentile range.

For example, review the average length of stay information for hospitals less than 100 beds in Exhibit 18–1. For the Q1 Year 2, Sample Hospital has a length of stay of 3.91 versus a benchmark comparison number of 4.06, a favorable performance against the 50th percentile by 0.15 (the –0.15 indicates an amount under the 50th percentile that, in the case of average length of stay, would be favorable). This performance places the hospitals score in the 35th to 40th percentile of all respondents.

As the CFO already knows, Sample Hospital is in trouble. In most cases, the facility is either at or below (worse than) the 50th percentile information. Most of the labor productivity measures are in the 60th to 65th percentile range, with the cost information in the same relative range. This indicates that Sample is spending more than the peer group for labor and supplies. The utilization statistics also present a dismal picture.

Each statistic has to be evaluated against what it means to the institution before a conclusion can be drawn. For example, the occupancy percentage for Sample is 46.36% versus the 50th percentile of 57.66. This places Sample in the 10th to 15th percentile range for the comparison group of hospitals less than 100 beds. In terms of utilization, the CFO knows that a facility should be in the 80th to 85th percentile range to use all of its assets effectively.

What other statistics should the CFO review to assure that a higher occupancy percentage is beneficial to the hospital? The answer is average length of stay. Sample Hospital has a length of stay of 3.91 (as discussed earlier), which is favorable compared with the peer group, but an occupancy rate that is 11.30% below the 50th percentile for the peer group of hospitals less than 100 beds. If these two statistics are observed in combination, one could say that Sample efficiently manages its patients, but just does not have enough of them.

Other statistics bear the same message. The hospital is not profitable, and much of the problem is because the cost of running the institution exceeds the availability of patients to pay the bills. In other words, all institutions have core staffing requirements, and within a certain range of volume, most costs are fixed. Sample has 100 beds in use while the 50th percentile for its peer group shows 66 beds in use. Sample's plant is too big for its patient volume. These circumstances can mean the hospital is heading for disaster.

So what happened to Sample Hospital? As you can surmise from the data, the previous year (labeled "Year 1" on Exhibits 18–1 and 18–2) was not favorable. Three years previous, the institution was losing money at a rate of over $1 million per month. The next two years showed improvement (even though the data still shows concern), and the improvement trend continued through the year labeled "Year 2" on Exhibits 18–1 and 18–2. By using benchmarking data (and a lot of other analysis), management was able to determine and address many issues that forced this facility to perform below market averages. By improving quality, managing costs, and controlling productivity, the hospital was able to stabilize its financial position. In addition, with creative management and attention to both clinical quality and customer service, the occupancy percentage rose to above the 50th percentile. Finally, the operating margin improved dramatically. In the first quarter of year 2, the margin was minus 3.18. By the end of year 3, results showed a positive margin of greater than 2.5%, a dramatic turnaround. Benchmarking assisted in this turnaround by showing management where the need for improvement was greatest.

Exhibit 18A–1

Benchmark Data Report
Sample General Hospital
Compared to Hospitals of less than 100 beds

	Annual Average Year 1	Q 1 Year 2	Current Quarter Benchmark 50%ile	Variance	%ile Range
Severity/Length of Stay					
Average Length of Stay	3.80	3.91	4.06	–0.15	35–40
Case Mix Index (All Patients)	1.02	1.04	1.04	0.005	50–55
Case Mix Index (Medicare)	1.24	1.26	1.19	0.07	80–85
Productivity/Labor Utilization					
FTE per Adjusted Occupied Bed	5.11	4.68	4.44	0.24	60–65
Paid Hours per Adjusted Patient Day	29.12	26.67	25.3	1.37	60–65
Paid Hours per Adjusted Discharge	110.53	104.19	109.5	–5.32	35–40
Salary Cost per Adjusted Discharge	$2,638	$2,510	$2,510	$0	50–55
Costs & Charges					
Cost per Adjusted Patient Day	$1,704	$1,608	$1,448	$161	70–75
Cost per Adjusted Discharge	$6,467	$6,282	$5,909	$373	55–60
Cost per CMI (All Pat.) Adj Discharge	$6,328	$6,041	$5,837	$204	50–55
Cost per CMI (All Pat.) Adjusted Patient Day	$1,667	$1,546	$1,408	$139	60–65
Supply Cost per Adjusted Discharge	$1,046	$968	$867	$101	60–65
Supply Cost per CMI (All Pat.) Adj. Discharge	$1,024	$931	$829	$102	60–65
Gross Charges per Adjusted Discharge	$12,987	$14,155	$12,536	$1,620	60–65
Deductions Percentage	0.40%	58.46%	51.04%	7.42%	60–65
Net Charges per Adjusted Discharge	$6,112	$5,880	$5,929	($49)	45–50
Net Charges per Adjusted Patient Day	$1,610	$1,505	$1,424	$82	60–65
Utilization					
Average Daily Census	43.15	46.36	37.69	8.67	65–70
Occupancy Percent	41.09%	46.36%	57.66%	–11.30%	10–15
Outpatient Charges Percent	53.15%	54.02%	50.14%	3.88%	55–60
Beds In Use	100	100	66	34	90–95
Adjusted Occupied Beds	92.2	100.82	72.05	28.76	75–80
Total Patient Days excluding Newborns	3,936	4,172	3,392	780	65–70
Total Discharges excluding Newborns	1,036	1,068	751	317	80–85
Newborn Days as a % of Total Patient Days	6.95%	5.40%	4.61%	0.79%	60–65

Exhibit 18A–1 (continued)

	Annual Average Year 1	Q 1 Year 2	Current Quarter Benchmark		
			50 %ile	Variance	%ile Range
Financial Performance—Profitability Ratios					
Operating Margin	−2.26	−3.18	1.95	−5.13	15–20
Profit Margin	−2.26	−3.18	2.06	−5.24	20–25
Return on Total Assets					
(Annualized) (%)	−2.37%	−3.58%	1.22%	−4.80%	20–25
Return on Equity (Annualized) (%)	−6.56%	−11.19%	4.61%	−15.80%	15–20
Financial Performance—Liquidity Ratios					
Current Ratio	1.28	1.19	1.9	−0.71	15–20
Quick Ratio	0.54	0.56	1.56	−0.99	15–20
Net Days in Patient AR (Days)	50.73	49	51.86	−2.86	40–45
Financial Performance—Leverage and Solvency Ratios					
Total Asset Turnover—Annualized	1.07	1.13	0.99	0.14	65–70
Current Asset Turnover—Annualized	3.21	3.65	3.57	0.08	50–55
Equity Financing	0.38	0.32	0.47	−0.15	25–30
Long-Term Debt to Equity	0.77	0.85	0.56	0.28	70–75

Exhibit 18A–2

Benchmark Data Report
Sample General Hospital
Compared to All Hospitals

	Annual Average Year 1	Q 1 Year 2	Current Quarter Benchmark		
			50%ile	Variance	%ile Range
Severity/Length of Stay					
Average Length of Stay	3.80	3.91	4.81	–0.91	10–15
Case Mix Index (All Patients)	1.02	1.04	1.14	–0.103	25–30
Case Mix Index (Medicare)	1.24	1.26	1.38	–0.118	30–35
Productivity/Labor Utilization					
FTE per Adjusted Occupied Bed	5.11	4.68	4.87	–0.19	40–45
Paid Hours per Adjusted Patient Day	29.12	26.67	27.77	–1.1	40–45
Paid Hours per Adjusted Discharge	110.53	104.19	134.6	–30.41	10–15
Salary Cost per Adjusted Discharge	$2,638	$2,510	$2,927	($417)	25–30
Costs & Charges					
Cost per Adjusted Patient Day	$1,704	$1,608	$1,530	$78	60–65
Cost per Adjusted Discharge	$6,467	$6,282	$7,284	($1,001)	30–35
Cost per CMI (All Pat.) Adj Discharge	$6,328	$6,041	$6,115	($74)	45–50
Cost per CMI (All Pat.) Adjusted					
Patient Day	$1,667	$1,546	$1,268	$278	80–85
Supply Cost per Adjusted Discharge	$1,046	$968	$1,250	($282)	25–30
Supply Cost per CMI (All Pat.)					
Adj. Discharge	$1,024	$931	$1,069	($138)	30–35
Gross Charges per Adjusted					
Discharge	$12,987	$14,155	$17,196	($3,041)	35–40
Deductions Percentage	0.40%	58.46%	56.31%	2.15%	55–60
Net Charges per Adjusted Discharge	$6,112	$5,880	$7,419	($1,539)	20–25
Net Charges per Adjusted Patient Day	$1,610	$1,505	$1,529	($24)	45–50
Utilization					
Average Daily Census	43.15	46.36	142.98	–96.62	15–20
Occupancy Percent	41.09%	46.36%	69.38%	–23.02%	< 5
Outpatient Charges Percent	53.15%	54.02%	39.64%	14.38%	85–90
Beds In Use	100	100	206	–106	20–25
Adjusted Occupied Beds	92.2	100.82	225.9	–125.09	15–20
Total Patient Days excluding Newborns	3,936	4,172	12,868	–8,696	15–20
Total Discharges excluding Newborns	1,036	1,068	2,506	–1,438	20–25
Newborn Days as a % of Total					
Patient Days	6.95%	5.40%	4.52%	0.87%	60–65

Exhibit 18A–2 Continued

	Annual Average Year 1	Q 1 Year 2	Current Quarter Benchmark 50%ile	Variance	%ile Range
Financial Performance—Profitability Ratios					
Operating Margin	–2.26	–3.18	4.45	–7.63	10–15
Profit Margin	–2.26	–3.18	4.66	–7.84	10–15
Return on Total Assets (Annualized) (%)	–2.37%	–3.58%	4.04%	–7.62%	10–15
Return on Equity (Annualized) (%)	–6.56%	–11.19%	8.46%	–19.65%	5–10
Financial Performance—Liquidity Ratios					
Current Ratio	1.28	1.19	2.2	–1	10–15
Quick Ratio	0.54	0.56	1.74	–1.18	5–10
Net Days in Patient AR (Days)	50.73	49	55.76	–6.77	25–30
Financial Performance—Leverage and Solvency Ratios					
Total Asset Turnover—Annualized	1.07	1.13	0.93	0.2	70–75
Current Asset Turnover—Annualized	3.21	3.65	3.48	0.18	50–55
Equity Financing	0.38	0.32	0.5	–0.18	20–25
Long-Term Debt to Equity	0.77	0.85	0.59	0.26	65–70

PART VIII

Mini-Case Studies

Mini-Case Study 1: Proposal to Add a Retail Pharmacy to a Hospital in the Metropolis Health System

Sample General Hospital belongs to the Metropolis Health System. The new chief financial officer (CFO) at Sample Hospital has been attempting to find new sources of badly needed revenue for the facility. Consequently, the CFO is preparing a proposal to add a retail pharmacy within the hospital itself. If the proposal is accepted, this would generate a new revenue stream. The CFO has prepared four exhibits, all of which appear at the end of this case study. Exhibit 19–1, the 3-Year Retail Pharmacy Profitability Analysis, is the primary document. It is supported by Exhibit 19–2, the Retail Pharmacy Proposal Assumptions. The profitability analysis is further supported by Exhibit 19–3, the Year 1 Monthly Income Statement Detail. Finally, Exhibit 19–4 presents the supporting Year 1 Monthly Cash Flow Detail and Assumptions.

When the controller reviewed the exhibits, she asked how the working capital of $49,789 was derived. The CFO explained that it represents three months of departmental expense. He also explained that the cost of drugs purchased for the first 60 days was offset by these purchases accounts payable cycle, so the net effect was zero. In essence, the vendors were financing the drug purchases. Thus, the working capital reconciled as follows:

Working Capital:

Cost of drugs (2 months)	$303,400
Vendor financing (accounts payable)	($303,400)
Departmental expense (3 months)	$49,789
Total Working Capital Required	$49,789

The controller also noticed on Exhibit 19–4 that the cost of renovations to the building are estimated at $80,000 and equipment purposes are estimated at $50,000 for a total capital expenditure of $130,000. The building renovations are depreciated on a straight-line basis over a useful life of 15 years, whereas the equipment purchases are depreciated on a straight-line basis over a useful life of 5 years. The required capital is proposed to be obtained from hospital sources, and no borrowing would be necessary. In addition, the total capital expenditure is projected to be retrieved through operating cash flows before the end of year 1.

So how was the proposal received by the hospital's board of trustees? They first asked for a small market study to test the amount of prescription sales projected within the proposal. When the market study results came back positive, the board approved the project, and renovations are about to commence.

Exhibit 19–1 Sample General Hospital 3-Year Retail Pharmacy Profitability Analysis

	Year 1	Year 2	Year 3
Rx Sales	2,587,613	2,692,152	2,828,375
Cost of Goods Sold	2,047,950	2,088,909	2,151,576
Gross Margin	539,663	603,243	676,799
GM %	20.9%	22.4%	23.9%
EXPENSES			
Salaries and Wages	192,000	197,760	203,693
Benefits	38,400	39,552	40,739
Materials and Supplies	12,000	14,400	17,280
Contract Services and Fees	14,400	17,280	20,736
Depreciation and Amortization	15,333	15,333	15,333
Interest	—	—	—
Provision for Bad Debts	25,876	26,922	28,284
Misc. Exp.	3,600	4,320	5,184
Total Expense	301,609	315,567	331,248
Net Income	238,053	287,676	345,550
Operating Margin	9.2%	10.7%	12.2%

Cash Flow			
	Year 1	Year 2	Year 3
Sources			
Net Income	238,053	287,676	345,550
Depreciation	15,333	15,333	15,333
Borrowing	—	—	—
Total Sources	253,386	303,010	360,884
Uses			
Capital Purchasing	130,000	—	—
Working Capital	49,789	—	—
Total Uses	179,789		
Cash at Beginning of Period	—	73,597	376,607
Net Cash Activities	73,597	303,010	360,884
Cash at Ending of Period	73,597	376,607	737,490

Volume			
	Year 1	Year 2	Year 3
Number of Prescriptions Sold	55,350	56,457	58,151

Courtesy of Resource Group, Ltd., Dallas, Texas

Exhibit 19–2 Sample General Hospital Retail Pharmacy Proposal Assumptions

		Prescriptions per Day	Annual
1. Annual Prescription Estimates—Rate of Growth/Capture			
Year 1	225	55,350	
Year 2	2.0%	230	56,457
Year 3	3.0%	236	58,151
2. Average Net Revenue per Prescription—Yearly Increases			
Year 1			$ 46.75
Year 2	2.0%		$ 47.69
Year 3	2.0%		$ 48.64
3. Bad Debt Percentage	1.0%		
4. Average Cost per Prescription—Yearly Increases			
Year 1			$ 37.00
Year 2	3.0%		$ 38.11
Year 3	3.0%		$ 39.25
5. Inflation Rates—Per Year			
Salary and Wages			3.0%
Other than Prescriptions			2.0%
Benefits as a % of Salaries			20.0%
6. Initial Capital Requirements			
Building			80,000
Equipment			50,000
Working Capital			49,789
Total			179,789

	Year 1	Year 2	Year 3
Gross Margin	539,663	603,243	676,799
Net Income before Taxes	238,053	287,676	345,550

	Year 1	Year 2	Year 3
Beginning Cash Balance	—	73,597	376,607
Net Cash Activity	73,597	303,010	360,884
Ending Cash Balance	73,597	376,607	737,490

Courtesy of Resource Group, Ltd., Dallas, Texas

Exhibit 19–3 Sample General Hospital Retail Pharmacy Proposal Year 1 Monthly Income Statement Detail

Return on Investment Analysis	Month 1	Month 2	Month 3	Month 4	Month 5	Month 6	Month 7	Month 8	Month 9	Month 10	Month 11	Month 12
Average Rx Sales Price	$47	$47	$47	$47	$47	$47	$47	$47	$47	$47	$47	$47
Average Rx Cost	$37	$37	$37	$37	$37	$37	$37	$37	$37	$37	$37	$37
Gross Margin	21%	21%	21%	21%	21%	21%	21%	21%	21%	21%	21%	21%
Scripts per day	225	225	225	225	225	225	225	225	225	225	225	225
	7.4%	7.4%	7.4%	7.8%	7.8%	8.3%	8.3%	8.7%	9.1%	9.3%	9.3%	9.3%
Business Days in the month	20.5	20.5	20.5	20.5	20.5	20.5	20.5	20.5	20.5	20.5	20.5	20.5
Monthly Scripts	4100	4100	4100	4305	4305	4612.5	4612.5	4817.5	5022.5	5125	5125	5125
Rx Sales	$191,675	$191,675	$191,675	$201,259	$201,259	$215,634	$215,634	$225,218	$234,802	$239,594	$239,594	$239,594
COG Sold	$151,700	$151,700	$151,700	$159,285	$159,285	$170,663	$170,663	$178,248	$185,833	$189,625	$189,625	$189,625
Gross Margin	$39,975	$39,975	$39,975	$41,974	$41,974	$44,972	$44,972	$46,971	$48,969	$49,969	$49,969	$49,969
GM %	21%	21%	21%	21%	21%	21%	21%	21%	21%	21%	21%	21%
EXPENSES												
Salaries and Wages	$16,000	$16,000	$16,000	$16,000	$16,000	$16,000	$16,000	$16,000	$16,000	$16,000	$16,000	$16,000
Benefits	$3,200	$3,200	$3,200	$3,200	$3,200	$3,200	$3,200	$3,200	$3,200	$3,200	$3,200	$3,200
Materials and Supplies	$1,000	$1,000	$1,000	$1,000	$1,000	$1,000	$1,000	$1,000	$1,000	$1,000	$1,000	$1,000
Contract Services and Fees	$1,200	$1,200	$1,200	$1,200	$1,200	$1,200	$1,200	$1,200	$1,200	$1,200	$1,200	$1,200
Depreciation and Amortization	$1,278	$1,278	$1,278	$1,278	$1,278	$1,278	$1,278	$1,278	$1,278	$1,278	$1,278	$1,278
Interest	$0	$0	$0	$0	$0	$0	$0	$0	$0	$0	$0	$0
Provision for Bad Debts	$1,917	$1,917	$1,917	$2,013	$2,013	$2,156	$2,156	$2,252	$2,348	$2,396	$2,396	$2,396
Misc. Exp.	$300	$300	$300	$300	$300	$300	$300	$300	$300	$300	$300	$300
Total Expenses	$24,895	$24,895	$24,895	$24,991	$24,991	$25,134	$25,134	$25,230	$25,326	$25,374	$25,374	$25,374
Net Income	$15,080	$15,080	$15,080	$16,983	$16,983	$19,838	$19,838	$21,740	$23,643	$24,595	$24,595	$24,595
Accumulated Profits	$15,080	$30,161	$45,241	$62,224	$79,207	$99,045	$118,882	$140,623	$164,266	$188,861	$213,456	$238,050

Courtesy of Resource Group, Ltd., Dallas, Texas

Exhibit 19–4 Sample General Hospital Retail Pharmacy Proposal Year 1 Monthly Cash Flow Detail and Assumptions

Depreciation	Years			Month 1	Month 2	Month 3	Month 4	Month 5	Month 6	Month 7	Month 8	Month 9	Month 10	Month 11	Month 12
Renovations	15	80,000		444	444	444	444	444	444	444	444	444	444	444	444
Equipment	5	50,000		833	833	833	833	833	833	833	833	833	833	833	833
Total Depreciation		130,000		1,278	1,278	1,278	1,278	1,278	1,278	1,278	1,278	1,278	1,278	1,278	1,278

Cash Flow

	Month 1	Month 2	Month 3	Month 4	Month 5	Month 6	Month 7	Month 8	Month 9	Month 10	Month 11	Month 12
Beginning Balance	$0	($163,431)	($147,073)	($130,714)	($112,453)	($94,192)	($73,076)	($51,961)	($28,942)	($4,021)	$21,852	$47,725
Sources												
Net Income	$15,080	$15,080	$15,080	$16,983	$16,983	$19,838	$19,838	$21,741	$23,644	$24,595	$24,595	$24,595
Depreciation	1,278	1,278	1,278	1,278	1,278	1,278	1,278	1,278	1,278	1,278	1,278	1,278
Borrowing	0	0	0	0	0	0	0	0	0	0	0	0
Total Sources	$16,358	$16,358	$16,358	$18,261	$18,261	$21,116	$21,116	$23,018	$24,921	$25,873	$25,873	$25,873
Uses												
Capital Purchasing	130,000	0	0	0	0	0	0	0	0	0	0	0
Working Capital	49,789	0	0	0	0	0	0	0	0	0	0	0
Total Uses	179,789	0	0	0	0	0	0	0	0	0	0	0
Net Cash Activities	($163,431)	$16,358	$16,358	$18,261	$18,261	$21,116	$21,116	$23,018	$24,921	$25,873	$25,873	$25,873
Ending Balance	($163,431)	($147,073)	($130,714)	($112,453)	($94,192)	($73,076)	($51,961)	($28,942)	($4,021)	$21,852	$47,725	$73,597

Courtesy of Resource Group, Ltd., Dallas, Texas

Mini-Case Study 2:
Changing Economic Realities in the Health Care Setting: A Physician's Office Teaching Cases

Improving Patient Care in a Changing Environment: A Teaching Case*

William B. Weeks, MD, MBA

CASE PRESENTATION

Bob Collins looked across his desk with an air of frustration. It was 9:15 PM; he had been in the office all day, had seen 47 patients, and had answered innumerable phone calls. His desk was piled high with the incomplete charts from the day's patients, and he still had about half of them left to complete. Bob knew that the challenge of the next several hours would be in keeping his patients straight. With some dismay, Bob wondered if he was providing the best quality care, as he tried to remember patient presentations, lab tests ordered, and treatment plans developed from hours ago.

This chaos was not what Bob had anticipated when he completed his fellowship in geriatrics 4 years ago. He thought that he would be able to dedicate a large proportion of his time to geriatric patient care, having an adequate amount of time in each encounter to assess fully the complexity of his patient's needs, and that he would be well paid for this specialized knowledge. He thought he had found such an idealized practice in a semirural setting.

For the first year, Bob's practice was what he had anticipated. The large majority of his patients were older adults, he averaged 15 patient visits per workday, he could charge a premium for his specialized knowledge, and he had Thursdays off. Bob was the only geriatrician in his area, which supported a population base of 22,000. Managed care had not infiltrated the area and represented only 12% of the market. Bob had no managed care patients, and 95% of his income was derived from fee-for-service indemnity plans. He had a 6-month waiting list for patients who wished to have him as their geriatrician—patients who would gladly wait the 6 months to access his specialized knowledge. He received consultation requests from both of the large group practices in his area— Group West and Group East—neither of which was staffed with a geriatrician. He had admitting privileges at the local not-for-profit hospital, a small community-based hospital with 60 beds and an in-house, multilevel nursing home. He did consulting work for the nursing home about 1 day per week.

However, because of an increasingly competitive market, things had dramatically changed over the last 4 years. After his first year in practice, a regional health maintenance organization (HMO) began

*Source: Reprinted from W.B. Weeks, Improving Patient Care in a Changing Environment: A Teaching Case, Journal of Ambulatory Care Management, Vol. 21, No. 3, pp. 49–55, © 1998, Aspen Publishers, Inc.

to compete aggressively for patients in the area. The HMO had an affiliation with an academic center 45 miles away, which housed a geriatric residency program and was staffed with numerous subspecialists, including three geriatricians, two geriatric psychiatrists, and a geriatric nutritionist. The local practitioners were clearly encouraged by the HMO to refer to the affiliate, but there still seemed to be enough geriatric patients who wished to receive local care. Bob's waiting list had dropped to 2 months, but things were still good.

However, the market for HMOs had become increasingly more competitive. There were now four regional and national HMOs in the market, dividing 62% of the patient population. This came as a result of three major employers in the area encouraging employees and retirees to sign up with a lower cost HMO plan. The two group practices in the area competed heavily for the HMO volume, now accounting for one-third of the population. The salaries of the practitioners in both group practices suffered as a result of withholdings and capitation.

The impact on Bob's practice was great (Table 20–A–1). He initially resisted joining forces with either of the group practices, as they each contributed to about one half of his patient load through referrals. However, within 6 months, Bob felt as though he had no choice. He had seen his geriatrics practice dwindle to the point where he needed the additional income from general internal medicine patients to support his lifestyle. He joined Group West as a half-time generalist, with the hope that he could specialize within the group as a geriatrician. He discovered that the volume per day required for profitability was so high that the complex geriatrics cases he initially took on considerably affected his productivity. In his first complete year with the group, he did not get any of the holdback/bonus for his HMO work. As a result, over the next 6 months, he attempted to trim his geriatric caseload by agreeing to see an increasing proportion of general internal medicine patients.

In addition, there had been a major impact on Bob's geriatric private practice and his relationship with the hospital. After joining Group West, his referrals from Group East stopped. Group East had to make better use of the academic resources available

Table 20–A–1 A Summary of Changes in Bob's Practice over the Past 5 Years

Bob's Practice	2002	2006
% geriatric patients	75	35
Number of scheduled visits per day	15	28
Overbooks	3	10
Waiting list	6 mos	3 weeks
No-show rate	8%	20%
AM	8%	35%
PM	8%	7%
Bob's net income	$143,000	$145,000
% of Bob's net income from indemnity plans	95%	30%
% of Bob's income from managed care	0%	65%
% income from Hospital Care Services	25%	6%

through its affiliate for referrals. It was clear that the camaraderie that had existed between the groups had vanished in the competitive atmosphere. Bob was also concerned that an additional geriatrician in the area would only increase the impact on his practice, as Group East might become more aggressive in pursuing the geriatric population. Although Bob had previously spent 1 day a week consulting to the hospital-based nursing home, he now managed only a few cases sporadically, generally patients who were not well covered by insurance or were poorly reimbursed through a state payment mechanism. The local not-for-profit hospital had developed an affiliation with the academic medical center, decreasing its bed capacity to 35 beds and eliminating one half of the nursing home. Selected demographic and economic changes in the region are shown in Table 20–A–2.

The complexities rose exponentially when Bob considered the actual seeing of patients. From a patient care perspective, Bob was concerned about the results of a recent survey that examined patient satisfaction with care (Figure 20–A–1). Of particular concern were the complaints of excessive waiting times experienced by Bob's patients. Before all of the changes, Bob thought that a busy waiting room was the sign of a productive, caring provider. Now Bob was confronted with the reality that patients were leaving his practice because of having to spend hours in his waiting room. He knew that he could become more efficient with the processing of patients, but it seemed that he often encountered the famous "doorknob questions." These complex, time-consuming questions were usually the primary motivations for the patient visit and were expressed by the patient just as Bob was leaving the room. Another problem was his no-show rate. On any given day, 25% of his patients would not show up or would be considerably late, usually because they forgot the appointment. This created a backlog because Bob had to "work the patient in" and catch up with patients who needed to be seen.

Bob's work life was challenging from a staffing perspective as well. Because Bob's private practice office was located in the same complex as Group West, he saw both his private patients and the Group West patients in his own office space. Although the original agreement had called for a 50/50 split in office expenses, Bob's private practice was diminishing. He was spending more time in the Group West practice to maintain productivity standards, making a 75/25 split appear more realistic. He supported one nurse practitioner from his private practice income, and he was provided one nurse practitioner from Group West, who was only

Table 20–A–2 Summary of Selected Changes in Regional Demographics over the Past 5 Years

Regional Demographics	2002	2006
Population of catchment area	22,000	25,000
Percentage of population over 65	14%	14%
Median income	$35,000	$37,000
Physicians per 100,000	205	167
Beds per 1,000	2	1.4
HMO penetration	12%	62%

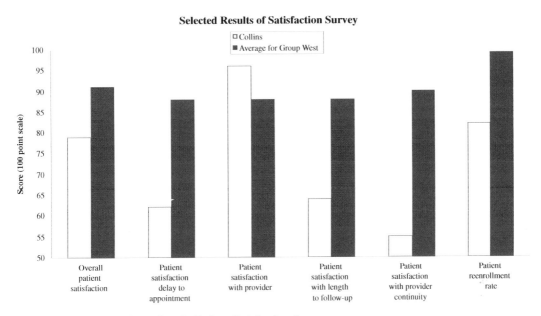

Selected Results of Satisfaction Survey

Figure 20–A–1 Selected Results of a Patient Satisfaction Survey

appointed on a rotating basis. Therefore, for most of the patients seen by the Group West nurse practitioner, Bob had to carefully review the encounters and be more available than he felt he should have to be. Most of this careful review came at the end of the day, after the nurse practitioner had left, leaving Bob to correct oversights on his own. There were problems with chart content and chart access, and Bob did not have data readily available about the plan to which a particular patient might belong. This became particularly complex since a number of the HMOs had launched Medicare managed care products, and the patients could change plans month to month but keep the same provider. Although Bob considered it unethical to treat patients differently based on their health care plan, it was evident that there were financial incentives that did not differentiate patient care but that did affect his and

the patient's income, such as which generic antibiotic was reimbursable to the patient in each plan or which plans would reimburse for which chemistry profiles. The result was that Bob tried to review the charts at the end of every day to rectify problems, taking an inordinate amount of time and generally resulting in few gains. He knew that his management of patient flow was not optimal but wondered how to improve it.

Bob was frustrated. His efforts to work harder only resulted in his spending more time at the office. He knew the system needed to be reworked, but he did not have the capital to automate all of the charts. He also knew that the population, given the referral streams to the academic center, could not tolerate an additional geriatrician without adversely affecting his patient stream further. After a quick call to his home to wish the kids goodnight, he returned to his charts, disgruntled, wondering why he had chosen the practice of medicine in the first place. What could he do to make things better?

CASE ANALYSIS

This complex case examines the impact of changing economic realities in the health care setting. Bob Collins' case is not unique to providers. Some of the problems in his practice seem obvious and easily solved; however, Bob is hesitant to invest even more time in the running of his practice, despite a realization that such an initial investment would pay off. The author examines the case from three perspectives and makes recommendations.

It is useful to consider the case from an "inside-out" vantage point. Figure 20–A–2 describes a conceptual model of health care. The patient and clinician perspectives are represented as "inside" the system, and external factors, such as government, business, and insurers, are depicted as "outside" the system. Bob's practice transformation has largely been a result of his response to external pressures: the changing health care marketplace and changes in the local medical economy. Bob may have little direct impact on "outside in" forces, but he has failed to respond to these forces in a productive manner. His focus has been from the provider and insurer perspective, almost to the exclusion of the patient or consumer perspective. Looking at the case from three perspectives and making recommendations for improvement will show how the "inside out" paradigm works from a consumer's point of view.

CUSTOMER PERSPECTIVE

Patients who are generally healthy and value their time probably would not want to be a patient in Bob's practice. A provider who

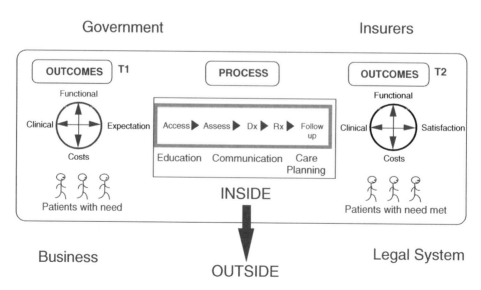

Figure 20–A–2 A Conceptual Model of Health Care with the Perspective of What Lies "Inside" and "Outside" the System of Care.

cares for a panel of patients under any type of risk system (whether capitation or bonus incentive) needs a mix of healthy and sick patients to have a successful practice. The inefficiencies inherent in Bob's practice are likely to create an adverse selection problem: the patients who are more ill, who are more reliant on the physician, and who may value time less will probably be satisfied with Bob—after all, he is a considerate, highly skilled physician. However, those who are less ill, are less reliant on the health care system, and value time outside the waiting room will probably seek another provider. Bob's inefficient practice style, with little apparent regard for patient time, will hamper him further because only the most ill patients will continue in his practice.

The lack of consistency among nurse practitioners would be an additional concern for patients. It would be beneficial for the patient to develop a relationship with a single midlevel provider. This relationship would improve Bob's practice efficiency as well because there would be less wasted time, as nurse practitioners would not have to review the case and history at each visit. The patient would value a personal touch— the recognition of the nurse practitioner who knew the patient and his or her case.

Finally, Bob could win patients if he were to add additional value to their visit. As is stated in the case, the Medicare HMO policies would allow patients to keep Bob as a provider, regardless of their plan choice. For instance, if Bob were to provide educational health maintenance videos in his office, he could provide valuable information, giving patients less of a sense of wasted time. Furthermore, the "doorknob" questions might be reduced, as the patient could gain information on "doorknob" topics without using as much of Bob's time. For the relatively small cost of a video player, television, and informational tapes, Bob could increase his patients' knowledge and improve their care.

ORGANIZATIONAL PERSPECTIVE

From Group West's perspective, Bob is a cost center. However, he may more than compensate for his own lack of profitability by providing valuable family services in a one-stop fashion. The value to Group West is Bob's geriatric expertise, his strong personality, and his ability to round out Group West's capacity to treat all ages. If Group West is like most other practices, it recognizes that engagement of the entire family leads to a more efficient practice and customer loyalty. These efficiencies are enhanced through the convenience offered to customers who do all of their medical marketing at one center, making the building space that Group West rents to a local pharmacy more valuable.

However, because of Bob's inefficient practice style and the changing mix of patients to a younger age group, Group West is losing most of Bob's value. Group West also faces a challenge from Group East, which is promoting its affiliated geriatrics expertise and may be recruiting its own geriatrician. Group West needs to improve Bob's customer orientation to maintain the market share and reputation it has.

First, Group West should provide a reliable nurse practitioner for Bob, making his practice more efficient. Second, Group West should offer to buy Bob's entire practice. Part of his practice difficulties are due to his management of the private part of his practice. This internal management is inefficient, and scale economies could be achieved through a single management of practices. Finally, after Bob's practice is integrated, Group West should leverage Bob's skill as a geriatrician more effectively. By targeting the entire family and promoting Bob's geriatric expertise, Group West could expect less "production" by Bob, improve customer value and loyalty, and maintain a family and community relationship and, therefore, increase profitability.

PROVIDER PERSPECTIVE

Bob appears to be miserable. He is frustrated by the rework he has to do as an inherent part of his practice. Until his practice system changes, Bob will continue in the same path, gradually losing his competitive advantage.

Bob needs to examine his practice from a customer perspective, both Group West's and his own. He needs to invest effort in improving patient care at a process level. He spends so much of his time doing rework that a minimal investment in process reengineering would have a terrific payoff.

Many of the suggestions from the previous sections would be important for him to consider. Of great concern is Bob's almost exclusive focus on his own bottom line. Customers pay for quality, even in health care. Within Bob's practice, the patients who are most ill clearly value him and pay with their

time. However, Bob is not leveraging the assets he brings to the practice. He should change his perspective from a focus on a stable income to a focus on enhancing value to the customer. With this focus, a stable income can take care of itself.

• • •

The author has presented a case and has examined the case from three different perspectives. It is important to note that customer value is a goal common to all three perspectives: the customer wants value; the organization needs to enhance customer value to remain profitable; and if Bob enhances customer value of the patients he treats, he can keep those patients. The case demonstrates the complexities of providing medical care in a changing environment. However, the case also demonstrates that much of the ability to enhance customer value rests with the practitioners and the internal systems managers. Managed care is not necessarily an evil force; many of the "evils" are poorly planned responses to a changing environment. The good news is that through a customer orientation, system redesign, and value enhancement, managed care can be managed.

Mini-Case Study 2:
Changing Economic Realities in the Health Care Setting: A Physician's Office Teaching Cases

The Anatomy of an Adhesion Contract: The Fallacy of Physician Choice in Contracting with Managed Care Organizations

Frank Welsh, MD, MHA

Adhesion Contract. A contract offered on an essentially "take it or leave it" basis without realistic opportunity to bargain. Consumer cannot obtain desired services except by acquiescing. Distinctive Feature: The weaker party has no realistic choice as to the terms of the contract.

Black's Legal Dictionary

Physicians worry about the percentage of penetration by managed care in their community with the attendant risks and responsibilities. Private practice groups and solo practitioners should be more concerned about the percentage of their own practice that has been invaded by managed care. What percent of patients came from each contract? Only by drawing up lists of contracts made and patients seen per contract as a percentage of one's entire practice can sense be made of where to begin with contract review and negotiation. Obviously, one large group practice that provides most of a town's care has more say in what it is willing to accept in contract terms than a solo prac-

titioner. For the solo practitioner or for the individual physician in his own group, any contract is an adhesion contract.

A leading payer's contract arrived on my desk recently with a three-week deadline to return it signed. The contract consisted of 26 pages of verbiage and a 17-page administrative guide. There were 43 single-spaced pages renumbered nine times; that is the first section was page 1 through 7; the second page was 1 to 2; the third, 1 to 4; the fourth, 1 to 4; the fifth, 1 to 5; the sixth, 1 to 2; the seventh, 1 page; the eighth, 1 page; and the ninth, pages 1 through 17. There was no table of contents so I prepared the following:

Should I renumber the 43 pages in order as stapled together? Should I read this contract work line by line or word by word? Should I skim over parts? Should I assume that some of it is repetitious? Should I hire someone else to read it and explain it to me? Should I join a group with a contract manager who reads all contracts from all payers for the entire group? Does it make any difference whether I read it or not? Is reading the contract really necessary? Financially necessary? Ethically necessary? Peace of mind necessary? Some form of off-Broadway entertainment? Yes. There must be some entertainment value in reading the contract.

Sure enough, among the rules of engagement proposed by the plan, two principles stand out. We are told that treatment must be provided if believed necessary by the professions, regardless of whether the plan pays for it, and treatment options must be discussed regardless of coverage. This approach is being forced on the plans by legislative authorities in recent years. Does this mean that the patients should also read their contracts line by line and seek fill-in insurance for "uncovered services?" Should the provider carry fill insurance for services that he or she provides and is surprised to discover are not covered? This is a risk of being a medical service provider in the current era. There may also be a risk of being a patient. Surely there must be someone out there to ensure against such a risk. Let us call this the plan's risk exportation cause. Is it negotiable? Certainly not.

The second encouraging word is that physicians should discuss any and all factors that could affect one's ability to provide care, including financial incentives with the patient. Full disclosure is encouraged now, but this was not always so. Not too many contracts ago, the plan forbade practitioners from discussing financial restraints, and that continued until enough lawsuits, national press reports, and media exposés persuaded plans to do otherwise. Let us call this the informed consent clause. How much informed consent is enough? There is probably never enough.

The contract itself appeared to be clearly divided into the responsibilities of the physician and the responsibilities for the plan and was couched in terms reminiscent of a boxing match or perhaps a duel. The practitioner must notify the plan of claims for payment within 90 days of services provided and, beginning one year from the acceptance of the contract, is to submit all claims electronically. But one might ask whether there is a comparable pledge by the plan to pay within 90 days. Well, there was not such a pledge from the plan without a law to insist on it—the prompt-pay law. The insistence on electronic claims processing was intended to reduce claims processing costs, but of course, this initially increases the costs for computer hardware, computer software, and training imposed on the practitioner. In an era of reimbursement restraint, these demands are hardly reasonable or fair.

Repeated throughout all of these paragraphs is the phrase "you may not charge the patient if your services are covered by their benefit contract, unless the services are not covered." We are at a time when the fewer services provided, the better it is for the practitioner, assuming patients want his services at his asking price. The plan makes no promise whatsoever to pay in a specific time frame except under penalty of the law. The plan does promise to pay the lesser of what you ask for or their fee schedule. Their fee schedule is invariably less than what is asked—thus the adhesion, the lop-sidedness. The plan can "update" a fee schedule at their volition; like "at-will" employment, it is not at will reimbursement contract with no practical recourse other than 90 days

notice of change. Furthermore, individual claims may be "adjusted" by the payer for a full year after payment, but other payors reserve the right to audit and change payments for five years, so getting paid and knowing what you can hang onto is unknown, in limbo, essentially indefinitely, unless established by law and not in the contract at all.

With regard to changing the contract, the plan can change the contract anytime with 90 days notice by sending out an amendment. No response, no signature by the provider is necessary. So, what is a contract, one might ask, if it is infinitely fungible? Although either party can terminate if it becomes insolvent, this strongly favors the plan that could file for bankruptcy and hold onto plenty of money earmarked for services already provided; the practitioner simply loses, thus again the adhesion. Sooner or later, a contract clause will be indecipherable or phrased in order to "have it both ways" and succeed in having it not at all. For example, plan payment methods may be explained to the patient, but not specific fees. This, of course, flies in the face of the plan's principal that "full disclosure" regarding financial incentive should be discussed with the patient. It should come as no wonder that a document this long and convoluted would eventually contradict itself.

Disagreements, likewise, are dealt with in a waffling way. The first paragraph states that binding arbitration will be used. The second paragraph states that if the dispute is litigated anyway (so what's binding about the arbitration?) there will not be a jury trial, as if this could be determined in advance. The contract does come back to deny any responsibility for healthcare treatment decisions echoing earlier denials, and in further denial, the contract may be sold like a home mortgage might be sold from one plan to another. Now management consultants advise that contract evaluation is an annual process, and if done regularly, it is easier and less time consuming then when first done; but this is true only if the contract content and format have stayed nearly the same. Contracts do not stay the same. To proceed, one needs a copy of the contract and a payer fee schedule. This is typically offered as only a peek at some fees, usually having nothing to do with one's specialty. This is where the dialog begins. Consultants suggest sending the payer a list of your two dozen most desirable and/or most frequently used codes and your charges. This list can be e-mailed in Excel format with the insistence that the plan supply their payments for each code. Dividing each expected plan payment by your charge for the procedure gives the percentage charge paid, which can be calculated for other plans and compared with the plan contract currently being evaluated. The format is as follows: a series of 25 different procedures down the left-hand side of the page, then a column for codes for each procedure, then your charge for each procedure, and then Plan A payment divided by my charge to give the percentage, which is usually 23 to 27 percent and so on for Plan B, Plan C, etc. (see Exhibit 20-B-1).

The plan with the highest percentage of payments/charges is worth sticking with, while the plan with the lowest percentage would be the first to go, unless it made up the bulk of one's practice.

Another way of looking at the plan is by listing accounts receivable by each plan. The plans make their money by investing yours rather than by promptly sending it to you. The longer they drag their feet in paying you, the better they do, especially in a more favorable investment environment. If one plan holds back all of your money for more than 90 days and another holds only 25 percent of your money for 90 days, you can easily pick the more desirable plan. These are aged accounts receivable. Of course, all of these analyses must be weighted according to how large a proportion of your business each plan represents. Thus, accounts receivable must be aged and weighted to determine their importance to your practice. State prompt-pay laws can help you reduce your days in accounts receivable and assess legally mandated interest payments, but this takes considerable extra bookkeeping on your part.

Payers who control 20 percent or more of a practice's revenues may have to be tolerated to avoid cutting receipts. Another way to look at the importance of charges to receipts ratio is to compare the percent of practice charges assessed to that payer with the percentage of practice revenues received. A payer may be asked to pay 20 percent of your revenues but may contribute only 10 percent of your receipts. The closer together these figures are, the more valuable the payer is to the practice; the further apart, the less valuable. Ratio analysis of a business's financial statements is widely used in the stock trading industry and by

Exhibit 20–B-1 List of Most Frequently Used Codes and Charges

```
Procedure [ Code [ My Charge [ Plan A [ % ] Plan B [ % ] Plan C [ % ]
1       Payment/my charge
2.
etc.
```

bondholders to determine what to buy, what to hold, and when to reinvest.

A study of explanations of benefits and a list of denials for payment can strengthen your hand in the appeals process. Knowing which codes are subject to unfavorable interpretation by payers will help you to identify payments worth appealing. Registered nurse, first assistance at surgical procedures can bill for 20 percent of the allowed fees. Bilateral procedures should be paid 150 percent of the allowed fee. Modifier 57 decision for surgery is paid for by Medicare. Modifier 25-25 may be used for evaluation in management services on the same day as surgery if clearly separate from the operation, and Modifier-51 pays at 100 percent for the first procedure, 50 percent for the second procedure, and 25 percent for each subsequent procedure done on the same occasion.

Can we providers sell our side of the contract, perhaps to someone abroad? Not likely. Although this first section concludes with the request for the physician signature "if you agree," it certainly does not give any procedural advice regarding what to do if you disagree. In other words, it is offered on an essentially nonnegotiable take it or leave it basis; thus, it is an adhesion contract—you're stuck with it!

The next page of the contract points out definitions, state regulations, an administrative guide, malpractice insurance requirements, and a fee schedule allegedly custom prepared for you but includes none (zero) of the operative procedures you do. Only office visits, emergency department visits, and hospital rounds are mentioned in a mere page and a half chart of allowances. E-mailing fees to the plan to compare with charges is now well understood to be a futile exercise if one thinks payments will change for the better.

The next three sections of the contract deal with state-specific requirements for providing contract services to residents in each of the three contiguous states. Because of dramatic differences in state malpractice insurance environments, fulfilling contract requirements may be prohibitively expensive in one state while marginally possible in another. For example, carrying medical malpractice insurance in the first neighboring state, described in four pages, calls for payment of a malpractice insurance surcharge into that state's patient compensation fund. This applies only if one sees residents of that state who are covered by certain of the plan's HMO products. The surcharge in my case is $14,000 annually, but the number of patients who fit the coverage criterion may be too few to justify this expense. Again, as the plan goes broke, the provider must still care for the patient for 60 days with no hope of compensation. Also, the plan can amend the contract 45 days before this taking effect in this state. Again, nothing prevents disclosing financial incentives—a permission mandated by law in state after state.

The plan's home state requirements are described in yet another four-page appendix. These are examples from my contract. Primary care must be available 24 hours a day, seven days a week. The provider shall not bill the patient, even if the plan goes bankrupt, and its services shall be continued for 30 days after bankruptcy in order to ensure continued care until new payment arrangements are made. All medical care plans shall be completed.

Whereas the physician practitioner must complete treatments without compensation, hospitals fare better. As large entities, they have, obviously, negotiated with legislature and with the healthcare plans to ensure coverage of hospital services until a patient is discharged or that care is no longer needed or that benefit limits intervene or that new coverage has been obtained. The physician gets no such protection from the law in this state. In addition to providing patient care complete, confidential records must be kept. Records subject to inspection by state and federal authorities are kept to ensure quality answers to complaints or for litigation purposes. These responsibilities may not be passed on to others by the provider without written consent by the plan. The plan, however, does not need to seek the provider's consent to sell its "block of business" to some offshore claims processor. Care shall be provided without discrimination or on the basis on an enrollee's participation in the plan (whatever that means). According to this, all comers must be treated, especially if they are covered by the plan regardless of how meager the benefit, if the provider is contracted to do so. The conversion of more and more medical care services into paperwork is insured by the legal protections for intermediary organizations. The healthcare insurance food chain is lengthened by fourth-party operatives that further intrude in the relationship between the principal insurer, the provider, and the patients.

To its credit, the state revised code mandates payment only 45 days after the plan received all "information necessary to process and pay the claim." This general statement is left open for interpretation by the plan and more than any other defines the fundamentally unfair advantage that the plan has over the provider. Plan administrators must stay up nights thinking of ways to keep changing the documentation requirements for a claim so that "all information necessary" is never well understood by the provider for long and is under continual revision. This maneuvering completely nullifies the 45-day rule.

Once again, the practitioner is left holding the bag.

The second neighboring state (B) offers a five-page appendix, little of which is not patterned after the home state and the first neighboring state, but bears close reading nonetheless. Neighboring state B goes for the throat with unreasonable demands should the contract be terminated, namely that care for enrollees with "special circumstances"—initially undefined—could be everyone—shall be continued for 90 days or nine months for the terminally ill or if beyond 24 weeks pregnancy through delivery plus postpartum exam at six weeks. Special circumstances are later defined to include disability, notoriously difficult to define in the ADA era, and congenital life-threatening illnesses—aren't we all mortal? Termination provisions are exquisitely detailed as set down in statutes because of past abuse of physicians by healthcare plans. The law now calls for notice of professional review action and reasons for taking action against the physician.

The right to have a hearing within 30 days is explained. It sounds more like a grand jury investigation, complete with notification of time and place and a list of witnesses against the physician. In fact, the hearing is an arbitration. It is held before an arbitrator and before one with whom the physician has no economic competition—as if one could be found. The physician is reminded to be represented by an attorney, doubtless to avoid coming to fist a cuffs with his accusers. A record of the proceedings will be made and available for sale to the accused physician, and the physician can bring his own witnesses, his own evidence, and present a written statement. If things go this far and the physician is a threat to the public welfare, the state licensing authority will be notified, and the physician's license will be suspended. Everything but the jury seems to be covered in these proceedings. It's a rough neighborhood, this second neighboring state.

The most galling provision of all is that the plan can negotiate "rates more favorable than rates between the doctor and other insurance companies." All of this is worded in a way so you cannot tell favorable to whom, although it should be obvious that this favors the plan and not the physician. Not too many years ago area hospitals howled mightily about having to match the lowest rates offered by any provider organization—so much for competition among big providers. Yet individual physicians would be pilloried for asking for uniformly high payments.

Next in order are listed the "products," insurance products, that is, that the doctor may choose to participate in, as described in an Appendix to the Appendix. Prompt pay and claims processing are similar to other state-imposed rules, so easily broken. The plan will disclose fees where discounted, as if they were not all discounted. Remarkably enough, subcontracting is allowed if it follows state regulations, but adjustments to claims are, again, open-ended. A "retroactive" denial of a claim may be made for an indefinite period of time. Fees may be provided, but only if requested.

Contracts include health maintenance organizations with and without a primary care physician, nonhealth maintenance organizations, preferred provider organizations, both with and without a primary care physician, contracts without networks, and Medicare benefit contracts. The provider "shall not take part in Medicaid benefit contracts or workers' compensation benefit programs." Shall not? This is literally the bottom line in the second neighboring state's state-specific regulations for physicians who wish to provide care for plan-cov-

ered patients. Is this restraint of trade? Is it the law of impossible alternatives? Is it antitrust? Is it poor wording? Apparently, neither the plans nor the physicians can be trusted to deal fairly in this state.

Medicare Advantage contracts call for yet another appendix, another two pages of single-spaced, small-font verbiage. This section "supercedes" any inconsistent provisions found elsewhere. Apparently even the drafter of these contracts ran out of time to check for internal consistency. Patient encounter data sent in with claims must be honest. Prompt pay by 60 days is promised. Balance billing is forbidden, even if the plan goes broke, although this does not apply to uncovered services. Obviously, if the plan goes broke, all services are uncovered and, therefore, presumably billable. Is this a light at the end of the tunnel or wishful thinking? Again, the current care and the current hospitalization must be continued without interruption and without hope of compensation until no longer medically indicated. The member (formerly a "covered life") is favored above all parties, and this is probably a good thing. To top it all off, the provider must immediately report to the plan if he or she is "disbarred." This is the first mention that doctors have been "admitted to the bar" in the first place. Is this attention deficit disorder or just good document drafting in the eyes of the law?

All records, premises, facilities, and equipment are subject to inspection for six years after the end of the contract while also maintaining strict confidentiality. In contrast to earlier provisions, subcontracting is permitted but is subject to all these same strictures. For good measure, yet another appendix is added to define the customers (the patients), the entities (the plan and its subcontracts), and their products (contracts for services). Finally, Medicare customers are defined along with a sobering statement regarding payment of the lesser of a physician's customary charge or a fee maximum determined by the plan less co-pays, deductibles, or co-insurance, doubtless to insure that all of the bases are covered.

As if this were not enough, a last-year's 17-page administrative guide follows. This guide helpfully starts out with how to get in touch with the plan and how to complete the 29 items needed to submit a claim. Also covered is how to ask for an adjustment if you felt underpaid (this would be all claims) and how to appeal a claim. Subrogation payments from other responsible parties and coordination of benefits get a mention. The specter of "retroactive change of eligibility" of customers is raised. The identification of customers and some products (six) as well as notification requirements for the hospital admissions, home health care, durable medical equipment, renal failure, and five surgical procedures are listed. Mental health and substance abuse services require reporting customers to the plan—so much for privacy where it might come in handy, although privacy would be regarded as enabling in some circles. "Care coordination," a kind of second opinion in advance, is called for to give an opinion regarding the worthiness of the patients to receive particular procedures. Recruiting community support for these benefits is included in the spirit of insurance generally. If the cost of care is to be widely shared, then the community or a representative of the community probably should weigh in on the worthiness of a fellow insuree to have certain procedures covered by the plan.

Providers are next identified as being part of a network of fellow providers who have also contracted with the plan. While unit cohesion is low among this fellowship of providers, documentation and record-keeping requirements are high. Providers are driven together by a common enemy, medical record details. No less than 38 items are listed in the guidelines for the complete medical record. A paragraph to a page of detail could be devoted to each of these items, leading the physician to spend a lot more time with the chart than with the patient. In an era when patients complain about physicians spending too little time with them, it is more important than ever to do the charting while sitting with the patient. This increases face time with the patient, even if attention is divided between the chart and the patient. Patients should be impressed with their care if they see the doctor meticulously composing their story and telling it word by word to the chart.

Of course, a patient's 12 rights and 11 responsibilities do not go undetailed. Whoever suspected there were more than ten commandments was right on target regarding the proper behavior of provider–patient interactions. Patients are also admonished to observe national preventative-medicine guidelines, an element of adhesion for them.

The penultimate administrative guideline does lift the tent to the possibility of provider plan dispute, and open the door to either informal discussion or arbitration, information available that the plan says is available on "our website." The administrative guide also has its own two-page appendix regarding Medicare Advantage—a 25-item list of do's and don'ts. Among the more adhesive clauses are those mandating the provision of certain preventive medicine services at no added cost to the patient whether included in the plan's covered benefits or not. Examples of these benefits are flu shots, pneumococcal vaccine, mammograms, and women's health specialists. The Centers for Medicare and Medicaid must approve your forms or brochures, and you must provide a language interpreter, training and self-care and ensure (sic) that subcontracting does not incentivise reduction in medically needed services. On top of all this, you must also comply with all the regulations of the Civil Rights, the Age Discrimination, the Rehabilitation, and the Americans with Disabilities Acts.

But if you have read this far, you may have wasted your time. Time is better spent analyzing receipts, billed versus paid, on a case-by-case basis, and comparing one payer with others.

Even then, past payments are no guarantee of future returns—unless the payer has been sued to pay out 100 million more dollars in the next three years, as happened to this payer. How to measure the payout? How to know when the payout is enough? There is no way to track this. It is simply a feel-good exercise as a result of a massive litigation effort. Is an adhesion contract better than no contract at all? Very little, when read in detail. The rambling construction, internal inconsistencies, and the impossible alternatives serve more as a springboard for contention than an affirmation of agreement. These features also explain why mass-produced adhesion contracts are so widely ignored.

Mini-Case Study 2:
Changing Economic Realities in the Health Care Setting: A Physician's Office Teaching Cases

Relative Value Units and the Physician Fee Schedule*

OVERVIEW

What does the Resource-Based Relative Value Scale (RBRVS) system do?

It ranks services in relation to the relative costs required to provide them.

How does the RBRVS system work?

The costs are expressed in term of units, known as "relative value units" (RVUs). Thus, the RBRVS is the payment system, and the RVUs are the units of measure within the payment system.

How do the RVUs work as units of measure?

The weight of the RVUs is "relative to" a measure of the level of effort against a unit of one. The comparable service used as the benchmark (a unit of one) is the midlevel clinic visit. In the case of evaluation and management visits, the higher the level of care, the greater the RVU weight. The weight for the highest level of care is about six times the weight for the lowest level. Other comparisons are presented in Exhibit 20–C–1.

COMPOSITION OF THE RBRVS SYSTEM

There are three segments of cost, each of which has its own set of RVUs. The three segments, or components, include the following:

- Physician work unit
- Practice expense
- Malpractice insurance

The physician work unit represents the time required for the physician to render a particular service. Practice expense represents the expenses incurred to provide services in the office setting, including such items as labor, supplies, equipment, office rent, and utilities. Malpractice insurance represents the professional liability insurance expense incurred by the practice. The three segments of cost are added together to arrive at the overall RVU total.

Exhibit 20–C–1 RVUs as Units of Measure

- RVU comparisons include the following:
- RVUs for new patients are higher than for established patients.
- RVUs for an initial hospital visit are higher than RVUs for a follow-up visit.
- RVUs for an initial consultation exceed the RVUs for a follow-up consultation.

---

*Source: Resource Group, Ltd., Dallas, Texas © 2005.

218

However, there is still another subcomponent of valuation to consider. That concerns where the service occurred:

- Facility
- Nonfacility

Facility indicates the service was performed in a hospital, an ambulatory service center or a skilled nursing facility. All of these sites are outside of the physician's office. Nonfacility, on the other hand, means a service that is routinely provided within the physician's office.

Within the physician fee schedule a different RVU valuation is assigned to the facility versus nonfacility location where the service is performed. Because the nonfacility RVU total represents services performed in the office, the RVU valuation will be higher. Why? Because services in the office will use more resources, this higher resource consumption is reflected in a higher RVU value.

Relative Value Weights and the Physician Fee Schedule

We now present a series of tables to compare and contrast types of RVU weights and to illustrate how RVUs are presented in the physician fee schedule. Since the tables are interrelated, we have inserted a line number on each for ease of reference. Also, the RVU weights used in these tables are for example only; in order to find the actual weights for the current year, refer to the Centers for Medicare and Medicaid Services (CMS) website first under the heading "Professionals" and then under the heading "Physicians."

Table 20–C–1 presents an example of total RVU weights for nonfacility and facility designations as we have just discussed. In Table 20–C–1, we see same procedure—an office visit for an established patient—with an RVU weight of 1.41 in the nonfacility (the office) on line 1 compared with an RVU weight of 0.95 in the facility (such as the hospital outpatient department) on line 2. As we have said just previously, services in the office will use more resources, so this higher resource consumption is reflected in the higher RVU value.

Table 20–C–2 presents an example of how the total RVU weights for the nonfacility, or office, are designated among the three segments of cost. You will remember that we have previously said each segment of cost has its own set of RVUs. Here, on line 3, we see the individual weights for the

---

Table 20–C–1 Example of Total RVU Weights for Nonfacility Compared with Facility Designations

Line Number	CPT*/HCPCS** Code	Description	Type of RVU Weight	Total RVU Weight
1	99213	Office/outpatient visit, established patient	Nonfacility	1.41
2	99213	Office/outpatient visit, established patient	Facility	0.95

*Current Procedural Terminology. AMA © 2004
**Healthcare Common Procedure Coding System

Table 20–C–2 Example of the Three Segments of a Nonfacility Total RVU Weight

Line Number	CPT* HCPCS** Code	Description	Pysician Work RVUs	Nonfacility Practice Expense RVUs	Malpractice RVUs	Non-Facility Total
3	99213	Office/outpatient visit, established patient	0.67	0.70	0.04	1.41

*Current Procedural Terminology
**Healthcare Common Procedure Coding System

segments: 0.67 for the physician work RVU; 0.70 for the nonfacility practice expense (PE) RVU; and 0.04 for the malpractice RVU, all of which add to the RVU total of 1.41.

Table 20–C–3 presents an example of how the total RVU weights for the facility or hospital outpatient department are designated among the three segments of cost. On line 4 we see the individual weights for these segments: 0.67 for the physician work RVU; 0.24 for the nonfacility practice expense (PE) RVU; and 0.04 for the malpractice RVU, all of which add to the RVU total of 0.95.

If you compare line 3 in Table 20–C–2 to line 4 in Table 20–C–3, you will see that the physician work RVUs and the malpractice RVUs remain the same; only the practice expense RVUs have changed between the nonfacility and the facility totals. Why? Be-

cause it requires more resource consumption within the expense of the physician's practice to perform a visit in his or her office than in the hospital outpatient department. Thus, the difference in relative value between the two practice expense values is logical.

Table 20–C–4 illustrates still another example: a code that is only applicable in on of the two care settings. In this case, we see a procedure—a code for initial hospital care—that has an RVU weight of 2.98 when performed in the facility—(the hospital) on line 6. We also see this code has an "NA" for "not applicable" in the nonfacility (office) care setting on line 5. Why? Because this code is exclusive to one care setting—the hospital. It cannot be recognized in the nonfacility, or office, setting. Thus, it is labeled as not applicable.

Table 20–C–3 Example of the Three Segments of a Facility Total RVU Weight

Line Number	CPT[1] HCPCS Code	Description	Pysician Work RVUs	Facility Practice Expense RVUs	Malpractice RVUs	Facility Total
4	99213	Office/outpatient visit, established patient	0.67	0.24	0.04	0.95

Table 20–C–4 Example of a Hospital Care Code That Is Nonapplicable in the Nonfacility Office

Line Number	CPT*/HCPCS** Code	Description	Type of RVU Weight	Total RVU Weight
5	99221	Initial hospital care	Nonfacility	NA
6	99221	Initial hospital care	Facility	2.98

Finally, Table 20–C–5 presents a comparative example of how the total RVU weights are exhibited in CMS physician fee schedule. On both line 7 and line 8 the layout shows one column for physician work RVUs and one column for malpractice RVUs because their RVU weights do not change between care settings. On both lines, however, there are two columns for practice expense (PE) RVUs: one for nonfacility and one for facility practice expense RVU weights. This is because, of course, the practice expense weights vary between the two care settings, as explained in the comparison of Tables 20–C–2 and 20–C–3. Then on both lines the Total RVUs appear in two separate columns: one for the nonfacility total RVUs and one for the facility total RVUs. Two sets of totals are necessary because of the variance in practice expense just explained.

Also note the distribution of the NA (not applicable) is in line 8. The NA that appears as a total on line 5 in Table 20–C–4 now appears in the nonfacility practice expense detail on line 8 in Table 20–C–5.

The Conversion Factor and the Physician Fee Schedule

How does the RVU weight translate into payment dollars? Through the conversion factor. The relative value unit that is expressed as a unit of 1.0 is assigned a dollar amount. This dollar amount is known as the conversion factor. For the sake of this example, let us assume the conversion factor is $40.00 for a unit of 1.0. (Although this amount is somewhat higher than the CMS conversion factor as this book goes to press, the even number allows for ease of explanation.)

As shown on Table 20–C–6, if we adopt $40.00 for a unit of 1.0, then an RVU weight of 1.5 would pay one-and-one-half times $40.00, or $60.00 ($40.00 \times 1.5 = 60.00$). Likewise, an RVU weight of 0.5 would pay one-

Table 20–C–5 Examples of Physician Fee Schedule Reporting of RVUs

Line Number	CPT¹/ HCPCS Code	Description	Nonfacility Physician Work RVUs	Facility Practice Expense RVUs	Practice Expense RVUs	Malpractice RVUs	Non-facility Total	Facility Total
7	99213	Office/outpatient visit, established patient	0.67	0.70	0.24	0.04	1.41	0.95
8	99221	Initial hospital care	1.28	NA	0.74	0.10	NA	2.98

Table 20–C–6 Conversion Factor Application

Line Number	Conversion Factor*	RVU Weight	Payment*	Notes
9	40.00	1.5	60.00	1.5 times 40.00 (60.00)
10	40.00	0.5	20.00	0.5 times 40.00 (20.00)
11	40.00	0.95	38.00	0.95 per Table 21.5 line 7 (38.00)
12	40.00	2.98	119.20	2.98 per Table 21.5 line 8 (119.20)

*Example only; actual figure will vary.

half times $40.00, or $20.00 (40.00 × 0.5 = 20.00). To use a further example, the 0.95 on line 7 of Table 20–C–5 would pay $38.00 (40.00 × 0.95 = 38.00), and 2.98 on line 8 of Table 20–C–5 would pay $119.20 (40.00 × 2.98 = 119.20).

Geographic Adjustments to the Physician Fee Schedule

Geographic adjustments to the physician fee schedule, called geographic practice cost indices (GPCI), are used to adjust for costing variations among different geographic areas. Separate geographic adjustments are made to each of the three components of the physician fee schedule (the physician work unit, the practice expense, and the malpractice insurance.) The adjusted results are summed to arrive at the dollar total. Tables 20–C–7 and 20–C–8 illustrate how the computation works.

As shown in Tables 20–C–7 and 20–C–8, the national unadjusted totals are adjusted to specific geographic areas by means of the GPCI. The GPCIs are published annually by CMS. The Philadelphia metropolitan area in this example (Table 20–C–6) receives an upward adjustment factor for each component on line 16 (1.020, 1.098, and 1.366). Each component's (physician work unit, practice expense, and malpractice) national

Table 20–C–7 Example 1 of GPCI Computation

Line Number	Example: Office/OP Visit, Established Patient CPT[1], Code 99213	Physician Work RVUs	Nonfacility Practice Expense RVUs	Malpractice RVUs	Non-Facility Total
13	RVU weights	0.67	0.70	0.04	1.41
14	Times conversion factor*	40.00	40.00	40.00	
15	National unadjusted totals	26.80	28.00	1.60	56.40
16	Times GPCI for Metropolitan Philadelphia, PA*	1.020	1.098	1.366	
17	Geographically adjusted totals	27.33	30.74	2.18	60.25

*Example only; actual figure will vary.

Table 20–C–8 Example 2 of GPCI Computation

Line Number	Example: Office/OP Visit, Established Patient CPT¹, Code 99213	Physician Work RVUs	Nonfacility Practice Expense RVUs	Malpractice RVUs	Non-Facility Total
18	RVU weights	0.67	0.70	0.04	1.41
19	Times conversion factor*	40.00	40.00	40.00	
20	National unadjusted totals	26.80	28.00	1.60	56.40
21	Times GPCI for rest of Pennsylvania (excluding Philadelphia)	1.000	0.916	0.806	
22	Geographically adjusted totals	26.80	25.64	1.28	53.72

*Example only; actual figure will vary.

unadjusted total (per line 15) is multiplied by its GPCI factor to arrive at that component's geographically adjusted total (e.g., 26.80 × 1.020 = 27.33, for example). Then the results on line 17 are summed to arrive at the overall total shown in the far right column of line 17. This amount (60.25) represents the final payment amount for the specific area.

While the Philadelphia metropolitan area's computation is illustrated in Table 20–C–7, the computation for the rest of the state is shown on Table 20–C–8. The mathematics of the computation follow the same pattern. Each component's (physician work unit, practice expense, and malpractice) national unadjusted total (per line 21) is multiplied by its GPCI factor to arrive at that component's geographically adjusted total (e.g., 28.00 × 0.916 = 25.64, for example). Then the results on line 17 are summed to arrive at the overall total shown in the far right column of line 17. This amount (53.72) represents the final payment amount for the specific area. In this case, the GPCI factors represent a downward ad-

justment from the national unadjusted total (53.72 vs. 56.40).

SUMMARY

Within the CMS formula, RVUs are set separately for each component of the physician fee schedule. The conversion factor serves to convert relative value weights into dollars. The geographic adjustment factor then converts these dollars into a geographically specific payment rate.

Other payers may use RVUs in a different manner. While some commercial payers link directly to the CMS RVU schedule, others may set their fees at some percentage of the Medicare fees. Some payers use the national unadjusted payment rates but use a different method for the geographic adjustments. Still others use the Medicare RVU weights, but set their own, different, conversion factor. Whatever the varied adaptations may be, the relative value system remains an important and widely used method for reflecting resource-based payments for the physician office.

CHAPTER 21

Mini-Case Study 3: The Economic Significance of Resource Misallocation: Client Flow Through the Women, Infants, and Children Public Health Program*

Billie Ann Brotman, Mary Bumgarner, and Penelope Prime

CONFRONTING THE OPERATIONAL PROBLEM

The Women, Infants, and Children (WIC) Program, a federal program managed by the county boards of health, provides a mandated health service under strict federal guidelines to women and young children. In this chapter, we analyze how a WIC clinic, located in the Atlanta metropolitan area, can serve its clientele more efficiently in an environment of constraints. We focus on achieving shorter waiting times for WIC clients through better management of the flow of clients through the clinic. We apply the peak-load framework from economics to this basic operations-research problem.

THE ENVIRONMENT

The WIC program provides nutrition counseling, limited physical examinations, and food vouchers for low-income pregnant women and for children with nutritional deficiencies who are five years old or less. WIC represents just one part of the integrated services provided to women and children by the county clinic. Other services include inoculations, medical visits with the nurse, and a variety of social services. Providing more than one health service at the county clinic is advantageous because it reinforces good health practices, provides intervention where necessary, and is convenient for the clients. However, it also complicates the management of service provision and makes it more difficult to improve the delivery of WIC's services.

To participate in the WIC program, a certification of income and health status is required. The first step for a client is to schedule an appointment for certification with a clinic nurse. Once certified, the client is immediately eligible to receive food vouchers and can return to the clinic to pick up her

*Source: Reprinted from B.A. Brotman, M. Bumgarner, and P. Prime, Client Flow through the Women, Infants, and Children Public Health Program, *Journal of Health Care Finance*, Vol. 25, No. 1, pp. 72–77, © 1998, Aspen Publishers, Inc.

vouchers for up to a year without revisiting a nurse. Vouchers may also be picked up when a client comes to the clinic for nutritional classes, which are required periodically.

From the providers' point of view, several activities directly related to the WIC program are managed simultaneously. They include the scheduling of appointments for certification, meeting previously scheduled certification appointments by the nurses, accommodating unscheduled clients who walk in seeking certification, and distributing food vouchers to eligible clients. (Eligible clients include those certified by the county clinic as well as those who have been certified by Kennestone Hospital and Home Visits, and Child Health.)

In principle, the appointment system is designed to regulate these activities. In practice, several factors, none of which are within the control of the clinic staff, undermine it. First, since clients come to the clinic for other services as well, they often are delayed for their WIC appointments. Second, of those that make appointments, 40 to 50 percent of them do not keep them because they either arrive late or simply do not come. Understanding the obstacles many of the clients face when arranging work schedules, getting transportation to the clinic, and arranging for child care, the clinic's management has instituted a policy of waiting 20 minutes for a client to arrive before rescheduling the appointment. Third, walk-ins are common and, according to federal guidelines, must be accommodated. In addition, the clinic has difficulty retaining qualified staff, and its physical space is limited. The end result is that women and children are often in the clinic for hours, are uncomfortable, and are unable to adequately care for their children during this time.

THE PEAK-LOAD PROBLEM

The economic problem faced by the clinic is one of demand exceeding capacity, leading to excessive wait times for the clinic's patrons as well as inefficient use of clinic nurses and clerks. The problem arises because the clinic's services are beneficial to the health of expectant mothers and children and are provided without fee to the patient. Without a price mechanism to ration demand, quantity demanded exceeds quantity supplied. This problem is not uncommon. It is encountered often in the public or quasipublic sector, when the price of the good or service does not adequately reflect the benefits of the good or service as perceived by the public.

In this case, the problem of disequilibrium between demand and supply is exacerbated by the fact that demand for the clinic's services is unpredictable. Clients often do not keep their appointments or arrive at unscheduled times. As a result, appointments may go unfilled, or two or more clients may seek the same appointment time.

On the supply side, capacity constraints, coupled with a persistent lack of sufficient numbers of experienced clerks and nurses, hamper the clinic's ability to respond to unexpected demand shifts. Moreover, due to employee turnover experienced by the clinic, few employees become sufficiently skilled to work as part-time clerks during periods of peak demand.

The economic significance of the problem is one of resource misallocation. In this case, too many resources are employed in the production of WIC services. The market solution is to increase the price of the service, thereby matching demand with capacity. But since that option is not available, efficiently managing demand and supply is necessary if the amount of resources used providing WIC services is to be reduced.

Federal guidelines for the WIC program leave little maneuvering room to improve the delivery of services. For example, the clinic cannot refuse to see unscheduled walk-ins; all clients must see a nurse for certification; all clients must attend nutrition classes; and vouchers must be closely monitored. Based on the data and information provided by the clinic, we determined that the fundamental cause of the queuing problem was the time spent by clients waiting to see clerks and nurses. Our hypothesis is that the flow of traffic through the clinic can be managed more efficiently by changing the current policy of waiting 20 minutes before filling a broken appointment with a "walk-in" to a new policy of filling the appointment immediately.

METHOD

We began by collecting information on the average daily client volume, the pattern of client flow through various services, the waiting points and times, and services rendered to the clients.

The data were collected by clinic personnel, recorded in a chart form throughout a day in periodic intervals, and included nine items:

1. Number of clerks available
2. Number of nurses available
3. Waiting time to see clerks for walk-ins and appointments
4. Waiting time to see nurses for walk-ins and appointments
5. Total time in the clinic for walk-ins and appointments
6. Waiting time to get vouchers

7. Number of nutrition classes
8. Number of appointments met
9. Number of appointments missed

The actual flow of traffic through the clinic is depicted in Figure 21–1.

Clients visit the clinic to keep an appointment with the nurse or attend a nutrition class or as an unscheduled walk-in. All clients first see a clerk to arrange for their records to be pulled. They then check in and wait to be called to their class or appointment. At the completion of the appointment, they see a clerk to pick up vouchers. Vouchers are also distributed at the end of the nutrition classes.

The General Purpose Simulation System for personal computer model simulates the average flow of traffic through the clinic. Estimation of traffic flow through the clinic is initiated when the client signs in and continues as the client meets with the clerks and the nurses. The model estimates the average amount of time a client spends in the clinic as well as average waiting times at each station. Clerk and nurse utilization rates are also generated assuming a variety of staffing levels. For comparison purposes, each version of the model is run with a 20-minute time lag before a late appointment is filled and then run with a 1-minute lag.

Six versions of the model are estimated using different combinations of numbers of clerks and nurses. Model A assumes that the clinic is staffed with three nurses and three clerks, Model B with two clerks and three nurses, and Model C with two clerks and two nurses.

RESULTS

Models A, B, and C present the results of all the computer simulations.

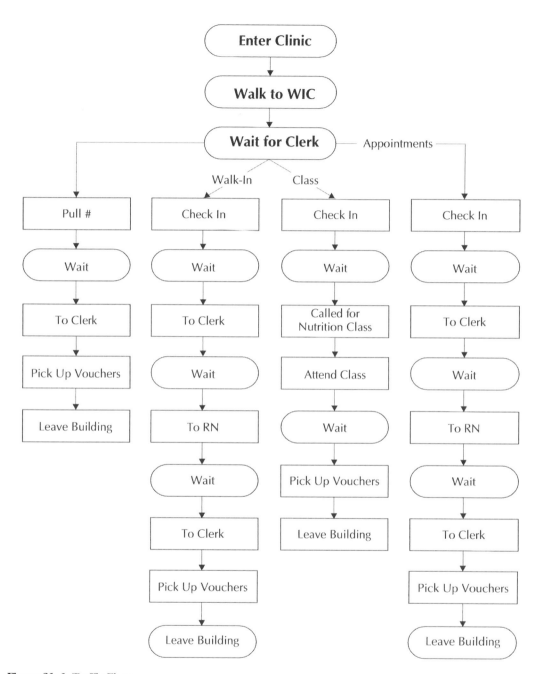

Figure 21–1 Traffic Flow

Model A: Three Nurses and Three Clerks

A comparison of the results generated changing a 20-minute wait to a 1-minute wait show that reducing the time before an appointment is filled results in the following:

1. A decrease in the total time in the clinic for the client from 3 hours and 16 minutes to 1 hour and 11 minutes
2. A decrease in the time spent waiting for the clerk from 1 hour and 9 minutes to approximately 3 minutes
3. An increase in time spent waiting for a nurse from 3 minutes to 10 minutes
4. A decrease in the utilization of clerks from 91.6 to 53.2 percent
5. An increase in the utilization of nurses from 46.7 to 61.2 percent

Model B: Three Nurses and Two Clerks

1. A decrease in the total time in the clinic for the client from 3 hours and 13 minutes to 1 hour and 27 minutes
2. A decrease in the time spent waiting for the clerk from 1 hour and 19 minutes to approximately 1 minute
3. An increase in time spent waiting for a nurse from 8 minutes to 43 minutes
4. A decrease in the utilization of clerks from 91.6 to 46.8 percent
5. An increase in the utilization of nurses from 51.2 to 73.3 percent

Model C: Two Nurses and Two Clerks

1. A decrease in the total time in the clinic for the client from 1 hour and 50 minutes to 1 hour and 9 minutes
2. A decrease in the time spent waiting for the clerk from 19 minutes to less than 1 minute

3. A decrease in time spent waiting for a nurse from 18 minutes to 13 minutes
4. A decrease in the utilization of clerks from 76.6 percent to 30.3 percent
5. A decrease in the utilization of nurses from 64.6 percent to 53.7 percent

In all three versions of the model that were estimated, the results of the simulations reveal that reducing the time before a late appointment is filled significantly decreases the time spent in the clinic by the client, on average, for all clients. Furthermore, the time spent waiting for both clerks and nurses decreases, the utilization of the clerks decreases, and the utilization of the nurses increases in two of the three estimations.

Greater decreases in waiting time occur when the clinic is staffed with three nurses and either three or two clerks. Smaller decreases occur when only two nurses and two clerks are available. This suggests that the clinic has little to no scheduling flexibility on days when it is understaffed, and a policy of filling late appointments immediately should be particularly beneficial.

The utilization of clerks and the time spent waiting for a clerk decreases in all three models when appointments are filled within one minute, and in every case but one, the utilization rate of nurses increases when appointments are filled immediately. This suggests that the flow of clients through the clinic is improved by filling appointments quickly. Utilization rates of nurses decreases only when the clinic is staffed with three nurses and three clerks. One explanation for this result is that the clinic is overstaffed with this combination of nurses and clerks. A supporting piece of evidence for this conclusion is that the change in rates of utilization for both nurses and clerks is the smallest when three of each are employed.

Another implication of these results is that if the clinic does not implement the expedited scheduling policy, it makes little difference to time spent in the clinic whether it is staffed with two nurses and two clerks or three nurses and two clerks. Both scenarios result in clients spending approximately 3.25 hours in the clinic. With the 20-minute wait before rescheduling, the clinic must be staffed with three nurses and three clerks if the time spent in the clinic by the client is to fall below 2 hours.

In summary, our results suggest that following a policy of immediately rescheduling missed appointments reduces the misallocation of resources employed in the clinic and thus permits the clinic to respond to its clients' needs more efficiently. Although this approach cannot duplicate the increase in efficiency that could be realized through the use of a price mechanism, it does improve the overall welfare of the clinic's clients. Filling appointments immediately results in shorter wait times for all clients, so no client is made worse off by the new policy. Moreover, as the patients realize that timeliness is important, more will arrive on time, further increasing the clinic's ability to monitor demand and provide services for its clients.

APPENDIX A

Checklists

Checklist 1   Reviewing a Budget

1. Is this budget static (not adjusted for volume) or flexible (adjusted for volume during the year)?

2. Are the figures designated as fixed or variable?

3. Is the budget for a defined unit of authority?

4. Are the line items within the budget all expenses (and revenues, if applicable) that are controllable by the manager?

5. Is the format of the budget comparable with that of previous periods so that several reports over time can be compared if so desired?

6. Are actual and budget for the same period?

7. Are the figures annualized?

8. Test one line-item calculation. Is the math for the dollar difference computed correctly? Is the percentage properly computed based on a percentage of the budget figure?

Checklist 2 Building a Budget

1. What is the proposed volume for the new budget period?

2. What is the appropriate inflow (revenues) and outflow (cost of services delivered) relationship?

3. What will the appropriate dollar cost be?

   (Note: this question requires a series of assumptions about the nature of the operation for the new budget period.)

   3a. Forecast service-related workload.

   3b. Forecast non–service-related workload.

   3c. Forecast special project workload if applicable.

   3d. Coordinate assumptions for proportionate share of interdepartmental projects.

4. Will additional resources be available?

5. Will this budget accomplish the appropriate managerial objectives for the organization?

Checklist 3 Balance Sheet Review

1. What is the date on the balance sheet?

2. Are there large discrepancies in balances between the prior year and the current year?

3. Did total assets increase over the prior year?

4. Did current assets increase, decrease, or stay about the same?

5. Did current liabilities increase, decrease, or stay about the same?

6. Did land, plant, and equipment increase or decrease significantly over the prior year?

7. Did long-term debt increase or decrease significantly over the prior year?

Courtesy of Baker and Baker, Dallas, Texas

Checklist 4 Review of the Statement of Revenue and Expense

1. What is the period reported on the statement of revenue and expense?

2. Is it one year or a shorter period? If it is a shorter period, why is that?

3. Are there large discrepancies in balances between the prior year operations and the current year operations?

4. Did total operating revenue increase over the prior year?

5. Did total operating expenses increase, decrease, or stay about the same? Is any particular line item unusually large or small?

6. Did income from operations increase, decrease, or stay about the same?

7. Are there unusual nonoperating gains or losses?

8. Did the current year result in an excess of revenue over expense? Is it as much as that of the prior year?

9. Did long-term debt increase or decrease significantly over the prior year?

Checklist 5 Considerations for Forecasting Equipment Acquisition

- Only one location?
- Equipment single purpose or multi-purpose?
- Technology—new, middle-aged, old (obsolete vs. untested)
- Equipment compatibility
- Medical supply cost
- High or low capital investment?
- Buy new or used (refurbished)?
- Buy or lease?
- Lease for number of years or lease on a pay-per-procedure deal?
- How much staff training is required?
- Certification required?
- Square footage required for equipment
- Is the required square footage available?
- Cleaning methods and equipment (and staff level required)
- Repairs and maintenance expense (high, medium, low?)

Wev-Based and Software
Learning Tools

HOMEPAGE FOR HEALTH CARE FINANCE

Health Care Finance: Basic Tools for Nonfinancial Managers, 2nd edition, has its own page on Jones and Bartlett Publishers' website. The homepage conains resources for instructors. The site can be accessed using the following URL:
http://www.jbpub.com/catalog/0763726605/.

OTHER WEB-BASED TOOLS

A user who prefers to use a business analyst calculator (as opposed to computer spreadsheets) can search the Web for a calculator distributor who posts an operating guidebook.

SOFTWARE TOOLS

Excel offers a series of computation aides.

Notes

Chapter 1

1. C.S. George, Jr., *The History of Management Thought*, 2nd ed. (Englewood Cliffs, NJ: Prentice Hall, 1972), 1–27.
2. C.S. George, Jr., *The History of Management Thought*, 2nd ed. (Englewood Cliffs, NJ: Prentice Hall, 1972), 87.
3. S. Williamson et al., *Fundamentals of Strategic Planning for Healthcare Organizations* (New York: The Haworth Press, 1997).

Chapter 2

1. J. J. Baker, Activity-Based Costing and Activity-Based Management for Health Care (Gaithersburg, MD: Aspen Publishers, Inc., 1998).
2. L.V. Seawell, *Chart of Accounts for Hospitals* (Chicago: Probus Publishing Company, 1994).

Chapter 4

1. Texas Medical Association, American Medical Association, Texas Medical Foundation, and Texas Osteopathic Medical Association, *A Guide to Forming Physician-Directed Managed Care Networks* (Austin, TX: Texas Medical Association, 1994), 3.
2. Health Care Financing Administration, *Health Care Financing Review: Medicare and Medicaid Statistical Supplement* (Baltimore, MD: U.S. Department of Health and Human Services, 1997), 8.
3. Health Care Financing Administration, *Health Care Financing Review: Medicare and Medicaid Statistical Supplement* (Baltimore, MD: U.S. Department of Health and Human Services, 1997), 9.
4. D. I. Samuels, *Capitation: New Opportunities in Healthcare Delivery* (Chicago: Irwin Professional Publishing, 1996), 20–21.
5. D. E. Goldstein, *Alliances: Strategies for Building Integrated Delivery Systems* (Gaithersburg, MD: Aspen Publishers, Inc., 1995), 283; and Texas Medical Association, American Medical Association, Texas Medical Foundation, and Texas Osteopathic Medical Association, *A Guide to Forming Physician-Directed Managed Care Networks* (Austin, TX: Texas Medical Association, 1994), 4–6.
6. C. Horngren et al., *Cost Accounting: A Managerial Emphasis*, 9th ed. (Englewood Cliffs, NJ: Prentice Hall, 1998), 116.
7. A. Sharpe and G. Jaffe, "Columbia/HCA Plans for More Big Changes in Health-Care World," *The Wall Street Journal*, 28 May, 1997, A8.

Chapter 5

1. S. A. Finkler, *Essentials of Cost Accounting for Health Care Organizations*, 2nd ed. (Gaithersburg, MD: Aspen Publishers, Inc., 1999).
2. G. F. Longshore, "Service-line management/bottom-line management for health care," *Journal of Health Care Finance*, 24, no. 4 (1998): 72–79.

Chapter 6

1. C. Horngren et al., *Cost Accounting: A Managerial Emphasis*, 9th ed. (Englewood Cliffs, NJ: Prentice Hall, 1998), 70.
2. J. J. Baker, *Activity-Based Costing and Activity-Based Management for Health Care* (Gaithersburg, MD: Aspen Publishers, Inc., 1998).

3. D. A. West, T. D. West, and P. J. Malone, "Managing capital and administrative (indirect) costs to achieve strategic objectives: The dialysis clinic versus the outpatient clinic," *Journal of Health Care Finance*, 25, no. 2 (1998): 20–24.

Chapter 7

1. C. Horngren et al., *Cost Accounting: A Managerial Emphasis*, 9th ed. (Englewood Cliffs, NJ: Prentice Hall, 1998).
2. J. J. Baker, *Activity-Based Costing and Activity-Based Management for Health Care* (Gaithersburg, MD: Aspen Publishers, Inc., 1998).

Chapter 8

1. J.J. Baker, *Prospective Payment for Long-Term Care: An Annual Guide* (Gaithersburg, MD: Aspen Publishers, Inc., 1999).

Chapter 9

1. S. A. Finkler, *Essentials of Cost Accounting for Health Care Organizations*, 2nd ed. (Gaithersburg, MD: Aspen Publishers, Inc., 1999).

Chapter 11

2. S. Williamson et al., *Fundamentals of Strategic Planning for Healthcare Organizations* (New York: The Haworth Press, 1997).

Chapter 12

1. B. A. Brotman, M. Bumgarner, and P. Prime, "Client Flow through the Women, Infants, and Children Public Health Program," *Journal of Health Care Finance*, 25, no. 1 (1998): 72–77.

Chapter 13

1. W.O. Cleverly, Essentials of Health Care Finance, 4th ed. (Gaithersburg, MD: Aspen Publishers, Inc., 1997).
2. C. Horngren et al., Cost Accounting: A Managerial Emphasis, 9th ed. (Englewood Cliffs, NJ: Prentice Hall, 1998), 227.
3. C. Horngren et al., Cost Accounting: A Managerial Emphasis, 9th ed. (Englewood Cliffs, NJ: Prentice Hall, 1998), 228.
4. J.R. Pearson et al., The Flexible Budget Process—A Tool for Cost Containment, A. J. C. P., 84, no. 2 (1985): 202–208.
5. S.A. Finkler, "Flexible Budget Variance Analysis Extended to Patient Acuity and DRGs," Health Care Management Review, 10, no. 4 (1985): 21–34.

Glossary

Accounting Rate of Return: See Unadjusted Rate of Return.

Accounting System: Records the evidence that some event has occurred in the health care financial system.

Accrual Basis Accounting: Revenue is recorded when it is earned, not when payment is received. Expenses are recorded when they are incurred, not when they are paid. The opposite of accrual basis is cash basis accounting.

Assets: The net value of what an organization owns.

Balance Sheet: One of the four basic financial statements. Generally speaking, the balance sheet records what an organization owns, what it owes, and what it is worth at a particular point in time.

Benchmarking: The continuous process of measuring products, services, and activities against the best levels of performance. Such best levels may be found inside or outside of the organization.

Breakeven Point: The point when the contribution margin (i.e., net revenues less variable costs) equals the fixed costs.

Budget: The organization-wide instrument through which activities are quantified in financial terms.

Business Plan: A document that is typically prepared in order to obtain funding and/or financing.

Capital: Represents the financial resources of the organization. Generally considered to be a combination of debt and equity.

Capital Expenditure Budget: A budget usually intended to plan, monitor, and control long-term financial issues.

Capital Structure: Means the proportion of debt versus equity within the organization. The phrase "capital structure" actually refers to the debt–equity relationship.

Case Mix Adjusted: A performance measure that has been adjusted for the acuity level of the patient and, presumably, the resource level required to provide care.

Cash Basis Accounting: A transaction does not enter the books until cash is either received or paid out. The opposite of cash basis is accrual basis accounting.

Cash Flow Analysis: This type of analysis illustrates how the project's cash is expected to move over a period of time.

Chart of Accounts: Maps out account titles

in a uniform manner through a method of numeric coding.

Common Sizing: A process of converting dollar amounts to percentages to put information on the same relative basis. Also known as vertical analysis.

Contribution Margin: Called this because it contributes to fixed costs and to profits. Computed as net revenues less variable costs.

Controllable Expenses: Subject to a manager's own decision making and thus "controllable."

Controlling: Making sure that each area of the organization is following the plans that have been established.

Cost: The amount of cash expended (or property transferred, services performed, or liability incurred) in consideration of goods or services received or to be received.

Cost–Profit–Volume: A method of illustrating the breakeven point, whereby the three elements of cost, profit, and volume are accounted for within the computation.

Cost Object: Any unit for which a separate cost measurement is desired.

Cumulative Cash Flow: The accumulated effect of cash inflows and cash outflows are added and/or subtracted to show the overall net accumulated result.

Current Ratio: A liquidity ratio considered to be a measure of short-term debt-paying ability. Computed by dividing current assets by current liabilities.

Days Cash on Hand Ratio: A liquidity ratio that indicates the number of days of operating expenses represented in the amount of unrestricted cash on hand. Computed by dividing unrestricted cash and cash equiva-lents by the cash operating expenses divided by number of days in the period.

Days Receivables Ratio: A liquidity ratio that represents the number of days in receivables. Computed by dividing net receivables by net credit revenues divided by number of days in the period.

Debt Service Coverage Ratio: A solvency ratio universally used in credit analysis to measure ability to pay debt service. Computed by dividing change in unrestricted net assets (net income) plus interest, depreciation, and amortization by maximum annual debt service.

Decision Making: Making choices among available alternatives.

Diagnoses: A common method of grouping health care expenses for purposes of planning and control. Such a grouping may be by major diagnostic categories or by diagnosis-related groups.

Direct Cost: These costs are incurred for the sole benefit of a particular operating unit. They can therefore be specifically associated with a particular unit or department or patient. Laboratory tests are an example of a direct cost.

Discounted Fee-for-Service: The provider of services is paid according to an agreed on contracted discount and after the service is delivered.

Equity: Claims held by the owners of the business because he or she has invested in the business; what the business is worth on paper, net of liabilities.

Expenses: Actual or expected cash outflows incurred in the course of doing business. Expenses are the costs that relate to the earning of revenue. An example is salary expense for labor performed.

Expired Costs: Costs that are used up in the current period and are matched against current revenues.

Fee-for-Service: The provider of services is paid according to the service performed and after the service is delivered.

Financial Accounting: Is generally for outside, or third-party, use and thus emphasizes external reporting.

Financial Lease: A formal agreement that may be called a lease but is actually a contract to purchase. This type of lease must meet certain criteria.

Fixed Cost: Those costs that do not vary in total when activity levels or volume of operations change. Rent expense is an example of fixed cost.

Flexible Budget: A budget based on a range of activity or volume. The flexible budget is adjusted, or flexed (thus "flexible"), to the actual level of output achieved or expected to be achieved during the budget period.

Forecasts: Information used for purposes of planning for the future. Forecasts can be short, intermediate, or long range.

For-Profit Organization: A proprietary organization that is generally subject to income tax.

Full-Time Equivalents: A measure to express the equivalent of an employee (annualized) or a position (staffed) for the full time required (thus, "full-time equivalent" or FTE).

Fund Balance: The difference between net assets and net liabilities; a term generally used by not-for-profit organizations.

General Ledger: A document in which all transactions for the period reside.

General Services Expenses: This type of expense provides services necessary to maintain the patient, but the service is not directly related to patient care. Examples of general services expenses are laundry and dietary.

Horizontal Analysis: The process of comparing and analyzing figures over several time periods. Also known as trend analysis.

Indirect Cost: These costs are incurred on behalf of the overall operation and therefore cannot be associated with the provision of specific health services. The finance office is an example of an indirect cost. Also known as joint costs.

Information System: Gathers the evidence that some event has occurred in the health care financial system.

Internal Rate of Return: A return on investment method, defined as the rate of interest that discounts future net inflows (from the proposed investment) down to the amount invested.

Joint Cost: These costs are incurred on behalf of the overall operation and therefore cannot be associated with the provision of specific health services. The finance office is an example of an indirect cost. Also known as indirect costs.

Liabilities: What the organization owes.

Liabilities to Fund Balance Ratio: A solvency ratio used as a quick indicator of debt load. Computed by dividing total liabilities by unrestricted net assets. Also known as Debt to Net Worth Ratio.

Liquidity Ratios: Ratios that reflect the ability of the organization to meet its current obligations. Liquidity ratios are measures of short-term sufficiency.

Loan Costs: Those costs necessary to close a loan.

Managed Care: A means of providing health care services within a network of health care providers. The central concept is coordination of all health care services for an individual.

Managerial Accounting: Is generally for inside, or internal, use and thus emphasizes information useful for managerial employees.

Medicaid Program: A federal and state matching entitlement program intended to provide medical assistance to eligible needy individuals and families. The program was established under Title XIX of the Social Security Act.

Medicare Program: A federal health insurance program for the aged (and, in certain instances, for the disabled) intended to complement other federal benefits. The program was established under Title XVIII of the Social Security Act.

Mixed Cost: Those costs that contain an element of variable cost and an element of fixed cost.

Net Worth: See Equity.

Noncontrollable Expenses: Outside the manager's power to make decisions, and thus "noncontrollable."

Nonproductive Time: Paid-for time when the employee is not on duty—that is, not producing. Paid-for vacation days and holidays are examples of nonproductive time.

Nonprofit Organization: Indicates the taxable status of the organization. A nonprofit (or voluntary) organization is exempt from paying income taxes.

Not-For-Profit Organization: See Nonprofit Organization.

Operating Margin: A profitability ratio gen-erally expressed as a percentage, the operating margin is a multipurpose measure. It is used for a number of managerial purposes and also sometimes enters into credit analysis. Computed by dividing operating income (loss) by total operating revenues.

Operations Budget: A budget that generally deals with actual short-term revenues and expenses necessary to operate the facility.

Operating Lease: A lease that is considered an operating expense and thus is treated as an expense of current operations. This type of lease does not meet the criteria to be treated as a financial lease.

Operations Expenses: This type of expense provides service directly related to patient care. Examples of operations expenses are radiology expense and drug expense.

Organization Chart: Indicates the formal lines of communication and reporting and how responsibility is assigned to managers.

Organizing: Deciding how to use the resources of the organization to most effectively carry out the plans that have been established.

Original Records: Provide evidence that some event has occurred in the health care financial system.

Overhead: Refers to the remaining expenses of operation that are necessary to produce the service but that are not directly attributable to that service.

Pareto Analysis: An analytical tool employing the Pareto principle, also known as the 80/20 rule. For example, the Pareto principle states that 80 percent of an organization's problems are caused by 20 percent of the possible causes.

Payback Period: The length of time required for the cash coming in from an investment to equal the amount of cash originally spent when the investment was acquired.

Payer Mix: The proportion of revenues realized from different types of payers. A measure often included in the profile of a health care organization.

Performance Measures: Measures that compare and quantify performance. Performance measures may be financial, non-financial, or a combination of both types.

Period Cost: For purposes of health care businesses, period cost is necessary to support the existence of the organization itself, rather than actual delivery of a service. Period costs are matched with revenue on the basis of the period during which the cost is incurred. The term originated with the manufacturing industry.

Planning: Identifying objectives of the organization and identifying the steps required to accomplish the objectives.

Present Value Analysis: A concept based on the time value of money. The value of a dollar today is more than the value of a dollar in the future.

Procedures: A common method of grouping health care expenses for purposes of planning and control. Such a grouping will generally be by Physicians' Current Procedural Terminology or CPT codes, which list descriptive terms and identifying codes for medical services and procedures performed.

Product Cost: For purposes of health care businesses, product cost is necessary to actually deliver the service. The term originated with the manufacturing industry.

Productive Time: Equates to the employee's net hours on duty when performing the functions in his or her job description.

Profit Center: Makes a manager responsible for both the revenue/volume (inflow) side and the expense (outflow) side of a department, division, unit, or program. Also known as a responsibility center.

Profitability Ratios: Ratios that reflect the ability of the organization to operate with an excess of operating revenue over operating expense.

Profit-Oriented Organization: Indicates the taxable status of the organization. A profit-oriented (or proprietary) organization is responsible for paying income taxes.

Profit–Volume (PV) Ratio: The contribution margin (i.e., net revenues less variable costs) expressed as a percentage of net revenue.

Proprietary Organization: Indicates the taxable status of the organization. A proprietary (or profit-oriented) organization is responsible for paying income taxes.

Quartiles: A distribution into four classes, each of which contains one-quarter of the whole; any one of the four classes is a quartile.

Quick Ratio: A liquidity ratio considered the most severe test of short-term debt-paying ability (even more severe than the current ratio). Computed by dividing cash and cash equivalents plus net receivables by current liabilities. Also known as the acid-test ratio.

Reporting System: Produces reports of an event's effect in the health care financial system.

Responsibility Centers: Makes a manager responsible for both the revenue/volume (inflow) side and the expense (outflow) side of a department, division, unit, or program. Also known as a profit center.

Return on Total Assets: A profitability ratio generally expressed as a percentage, this is a broad measure of profitability in common use. Computed by dividing earnings before interest and taxes, or EBIT, by total assets. This ratio is known by its acronym EBIT in credit analysis circles.

Revenue: Actual or expected cash inflows due to the organization's major business. Revenues are amounts earned in the course of doing business. In the case of health care, revenues are mostly earned by rendering services to patients.

Revenue Amount: Refers to how much each payer is expected to pay for the service and/or drug or device.

Revenue Sources: Refers to how many payers will pay for the service and/or drug and device and in what proportion.

Revenue Type: A designation as to whether, for example, revenue is derived entirely from services or whether part of the revenue is derived from drugs and devices.

Semifixed Cost: Those costs that stay fixed for a time when activity levels or volume of operations change, rises will occur, but not in direct proportion.

Semivariable Cost: Those costs that vary when activity levels or volume of operations change, but not in direct proportion. A supervisor's salary is an example of a semivariable cost.

Solvency Ratios: Ratios that reflect the ability of the organization to pay the annual interest and principal obligations on its long-term debt. These ratios determine ability to "be solvent."

Space Occupancy: Within the context of a forecast or projection, refers to the overall cost of occupying the space required for the service or procedure. Considered to be an indirect cost.

Staffing: A term that means the assigning of staff to fill scheduled positions.

Statement of Cash Flows: One of the four basic statements, this statement reports the current period cash flow by taking the accrual basis statements and converting them to an effective cash flow. This is accomplished by a series of reconciling adjustments that account for the noncash amounts.

Statement of Fund Balance/Net Worth: One of the four basic statements, this statement reports the excess of revenue over expenses (or vice-versa) for the period as the excess flows into equity (or reduces equity, in the case of a loss for the period).

Statement of Revenue and Expense: One of the four basic financial statements, this statement reports the inflow of revenue and the outflow of expense over a stated period of time. The net result is also reported, either as excess of revenue over expense or, in the case of a loss for the period, excess of expense over revenue.

Static Budget: A budget based on a single level of operations, or volume. After approved and finalized, the single level of operations (volume) is never adjusted; thus, the budget is "static" or unchanging.

Subsidiary Journals: Documents that contain specific sets of transactions and that support the general ledger.

Subsidiary Reports: Reports that support, and thus are subsidiary to, the four major financial statements.

Supplies: Within the context of a forecast or

projection, refers to the necessary supplies that are required to perform a procedure or service. Considered to be a direct expense.

Support Services Expenses: This type of expense provides support to both general services expenses and to operations expenses. It is necessary for support, but it is neither directly related to patient care nor is it a service necessary to maintain the patient. Examples of support services are insurance and payroll taxes.

Time Value of Money: The present value concept, which is that the value of a dollar today is more than the value of a dollar in the future.

Three-Variance Method: A method of variance analysis that compares volume variance to use (or quantity) variance and to spending (or price) variance.

Trend Analysis: The process of comparing and analyzing figures over several time periods. Also known as horizontal analysis.

Trial Balance: A document used to balance the general ledger accounts and to produce financial statements.

Two-Variance Method: A method of variance analysis that compares volume variance to budgeted costs (defined as standard hours for actual production)—thus the "two-variance" method.

Unadjusted Rate of Return: An unsophisticated return on investment method, the answer for which is an estimate containing no precision.

Unexpired Costs: Costs that are not yet used up and will be matched against future revenues.

Variable Cost: Those costs that vary in direct proportion to changes in activity levels of volume of operations. Food for meal preparation is an example of variable cost.

Variance Analysis: A variance is the difference between standard and actual prices and quantities. Variance analysis analyzes these differences.

Vertical Analysis: A process of converting dollar amounts to percentages to put information on the same relative basis. Also known as common sizing.

Voluntary Organization: Indicates the taxable status of the organization. A voluntary (or nonprofit) organization is exempt from paying income taxes.

Examples and Exercises, Supplemental Materials, and Solutions

The following examples and exercises include examples, practice exercises, and assignment exercises. Solutions to the practice exercises are found at the end of this section. Exercises are designated by chapter number.

EXAMPLES AND EXERCISES

CHAPTER 1

Assignment Exercise 1–1

Review the chapter text about types of organizations and examine the list in Exhibit 1–1.

Required

1. Obtain listings of health care organizations from the yellow pages of a telephone book.
2. Set up a work sheet listing the classifications of organizations found in Exhibit 1–1.
3. Enter the organizations you found in the yellow pages onto the work sheet.
4. For each organization indicate the type of organization.
5. If some cannot be identified by type, comment on what you would expect them to be; that is, proprietary, voluntary, or government owned.

Assignment Exercise 1–2

Review the chapter text about organization charts. Also examine the organization charts appearing in Figures 1–2 and 1–3.

Required

1. Refer to the Metropolis Health System (MHS) case study appearing in Chapter 18. Read about the various types of services offered by MHS.
2. The MHS organization chart has seven major areas of responsibility, each headed by a senior vice president. Select one of the seven areas and design additional levels of

detail that indicate the managers. If you have considerable detail you may choose one department (such as ambulatory operations) instead of the entire area of responsibility for that senior vice president.

3. Do you believe your design of the detailed organization chart indicates centralized or decentralized lines of authority for decision making? Can you explain your approach in one to two sentences?

CHAPTER 2

Assignment Exercise 2–1: Health System Flowsheets

Review the chapter text about information flow and Figures 2–2 and 2–3.

Required

1. Find an information flowsheet from a health care organization. It can be from a published source or from an actual organization.
2. Based on this flowsheet, comment on what the structure of the organization's information system appears to be.
3. If you were a manager (at this organization), would you want to change the structure? If so, why? If not, why not?

Assignment Exercise 2–2: Chart of Accounts

Review the chapter text about the chart of accounts and how it is a map of the company elements. Also review Exhibits 2–1, 2–2, and 2–3.

Required

1. Find an excerpt from a health care organization's chart of accounts. It can be from a published source or from an actual organization.
2. Based on this chart of accounts excerpt, comment on what the structure of the organization's reporting system appears to be.
3. If you were a manager (at this organization), would you want to change the system? If so, why? If not, why not?

CHAPTER 3

Example 3A: Assets and Liabilities

Study the chapter text concerning examples of assets and liabilities. Is the difference between short-term and long-term assets and liabilities clear to you?

Practice Exercise 3–I

Place an "X" in the appropriate classification for each balance sheet item listed below.

	Short-Term Asset	*Long-Term Asset*	*Short-Term Liability*	*Long-Term Liability*
Payroll taxes due				
Accounts receivable				
Land				
Mortgage payable (non-current)				
Buildings				
Note payable (due in 24 months)				
Inventory				
Accounts payable				
Cash on hand				

Assignment Exercise 3–1: Balance Sheet

Locate a health care-related balance sheet. The source of the balance sheet can be internal (within a health care facility of some type) or external (from a published article or from a company's annual report, for example). Write your impressions and/or comments about the assets, liabilities and net worth found on your balance sheet. Would you have preferred more detail in this statement? If so, why?

Assignment Exercise 3–2: Balance Sheet

Locate a second health care-related balance sheet. Again, the source of the balance sheet can be either internal or external. Compare the balance sheet you acquired for Assignment Exercise 3-1 with the second balance sheet you have now obtained. What is the same? What is different? Which one do you find more informative? Why?

CHAPTER 4

Example 4A: Contractual Allowances

Contractual allowances represent the difference between the full established rate and the agreed-upon contractual rate that will be paid. An example was given in the text of Chapter 4 by which the hospital's full established rate for a certain procedure is $100, but Giant Health Plan has negotiated a managed care contract whereby the plan pays only $90 for that procedure. The contractual allowance is $10 ($100 less $90 = $10). Assume instead that Near-By Health Plan has negotiated its own managed care contract whereby this plan pays $95 for that procedure. In this case the contractual allowance is $5 ($100 less $95 = $5).

Assignment Exercise 4–1: Contractual Allowances

Physician Office Revenue for Visit Code 99214 has a full established rate of $72.00. Of ten different payers, there are nine different contracted rates, as follows:

Payer	Contracted Rate
FHP	$35.70
HPHP	58.85
MC	54.90
UND	60.40
CCN	70.20
MO	70.75
CGN	10.00
PRU	54.90
PHCS	50.00
ANA	45.00

Rates for illustration only.

Required

1. Set up a work sheet with four columns: *Payer, Full Rate, Contracted Rate,* and *Contractual Allowance.*
2. For each payer, enter the full rate and the contracted rate.
3. For each payer, compute the contractual allowance.

The first payer has been computed below:

Payer	Full Rate	(less)	Contracted Rate	=	Contractual Allowance
FHP	$72.00		$35.70		$36.30

Example 4B: Revenue Sources and Grouping Revenue

Sources of health care revenue are often grouped by payer. Thus services might be grouped as follows:

Revenue from the Medicare Program (payer = Medicare)
Revenue from the Medicaid Program (payer = Medicaid)
Revenue from Blue Cross Blue Shield (payer = Commercial Insurance)

or

Revenue from Blue Cross Blue Shield (payer = Managed Care Contract)

Assignment Exercise 4–2: Revenue Sources and Grouping Revenue

The Metropolis Health System has revenue sources from operations, donations, and interest income. The revenue from operations is primarily received for services. MHS groups its revenue first by cost center. Within each cost center the services revenue is then grouped by payer.

Required

1. Set up a work sheet with individual columns across the top for six revenue sources (payers): *Medicare, Medicaid, Other Public Programs, Patients, Commercial Insurance*, and *Managed Care Contracts*.
2. Certain situations concerning the Intensive Care Unit and the Laboratory are described below.

    Set up six vertical line items on your work sheet, numbered (1) through (6). Six situations are described below. For each of the six situations, indicate its number (1 through 6) and enter the appropriate cost center (either Intensive Care Unit or Laboratory). Then place an X in the column(s) that represents the correct revenue source(s) for the item. The six situations are as follows:

    (1)   ICU stay billed to employee's insurance program.
    (2)   Lab test paid for by an individual.
    (3)   Pathology work performed for the state.
    (4)   ICU stay billed to member's health plan.
    (5)   ICU stay billed for Medicare beneficiary.
    (6)   Series of allergy tests run for eligible Medicaid beneficiary.

Headings for your work sheet:

	Medicare	Medicaid	Other Public Programs	Patients	Commercial Insurance	Managed Care Contracts
(1)						
(2)						
(3)						
(4)						
(5)						
(6)						

CHAPTER 5

Example 5A: Grouping Expenses by Cost Center

Cost centers are one method of grouping expenses. For example, a nursing home may consider the Admitting Department as a cost center. In that case the expenses grouped under the Admitting Department cost center may include:

- Administrative and Clerical Salaries
- Admitting Supplies
- Dues
- Periodicals and Books
- Employee Education
- Purchased Maintenance

Practice Exercise 5–I: Grouping Expenses by Cost Center

The Metropolis Health System groups expenses for the Intensive Care Unit into its own cost center. Laboratory expenses and Laundry expenses are likewise grouped into their own cost centers.

Required

1. Set up a work sheet with individual columns across the top for the three cost centers: *Intensive Care Unit, Laboratory,* and *Laundry.*
2. Indicate the appropriate cost center for each of the following expenses:
   - Drugs Requisitioned
   - Pathology Supplies
   - Detergents and Bleach
   - Nursing Salaries
   - Clerical Salaries
   - Uniforms (for Laundry Aides)
   - Repairs (parts for microscopes)
     (Hint: One of the expenses will apply to more than one cost center.)

Headings for your worksheet:

| *Intensive Care Unit* | *Laboratoy* | *Laundry* |

Assignment Exercise 5–1: Grouping Expenses by Cost Center

The Metropolis Health System's Rehabilitation and Wellness Center offers outpatient therapy and return-to-work services plus cardiac and pulmonary rehabilitation to get people back to a normal way of living. The Rehabilitation and Wellness Center expenses include the following:

- Nursing Salaries
- Physical Therapist Salaries
- Occupational Therapist Salaries
- Cardiac Rehab Salaries
- Pulmonary Rehab Salaries
- Patient Education Coordinator Salary
- Nursing Supplies
- Physical Therapist Supplies

- Occupational Therapist Supplies
- Cardiac Rehab Supplies
- Pulmonary Rehab Supplies
- Training Supplies
- Clerical Office Supplies
- Employee Education

Required

1. Decide how many cost centers should be used for the above expenses at the Center.
2. Set up a work sheet with individual columns across the top for the cost centers you have chosen.
3. For each of the expenses listed above, indicate to which of your cost centers it should be assigned.

Example 5B

Study the chapter text concerning grouping expenses by diagnoses and procedures. Refer to Exhibits 5–3 and 5–4 (about Major Diagnostic Categories), Exhibit 5–5 (about DRGs and MDCs), and Table 5–1 (about Procedure Codes) for examples of different ways to group expenses by diagnoses and procedures.

Assignment Exercise 5–2

Required

Find a listing of expenses by diagnosis or by procedure. The source of the list can be internal (within a health care facility of some type) or external (such as a published article, report, or survey). Comment upon whether you believe the expense grouping used is appropriate. Would you have grouped the expenses in another way?

CHAPTER 6

Example 6A: Direct and Indirect Costs

Review the chapter text regarding direct and indirect costs. In particular review the example of freestanding dialysis center direct costs (Exhibit 6–1) and indirect costs (Exhibit 6–2). Remember that indirect costs are shared and are sometimes called joint costs or common costs. Because such costs are shared they must be allocated. Also, remember that one test of a direct cost is to ask: "If the operating unit (such as a department) did not exist, would this cost not be in existence?"

Practice Exercise 6–I: Identifying Direct and Indirect Costs

Make a worksheet with two columns labeled: *Direct Cost* and *Indirect Cost*. Place each of the following items in the appropriate column:

- Managed care marketing expense
- Real estate taxes
- Liability insurance
- Clinic telephone expense
- Utilities (for the entire facility)
- Emergency room medical supplies

Assignment Exercise 6–1: Allocating Indirect Costs

Study Table 6–1, Example of Radiology Departments Direct and Indirect Cost Totals, and Table 6–2, Example of Indirect Costs Allocated to Radiology Departments, and review the chapter text describing how the indirect cost is allocated. This assignment will change the allocation bases: A) Volumes, B) Direct Costs, and C) Number of Films.

Required

1. Compute the costs allocated to cost centers #557, 558, 559, 560, and 561 using the new allocation bases shown below. Use a worksheet replicating the set up in Table 6–2. Total the new results.

   The new allocation bases are:

A) Volumes	120,000	130,000	70,000	110,000	70,000	500,000
B) Direct costs	$1,100,000	$700,000	$1,300,000	$1,600,000	$1,300,000	$6,000,000
C) No. of films	400,000	20,000	55,000	25,000	20,000	520,000

2. Using a worksheet replicating the set up in Table 6–1, enter the new direct cost and the new totals for indirect costs resulting from your work. Total the new results.

Practice Exercise 6–II: Responsibility Centers

The Metropolis Health System has one Director who supervises the areas of Security, Communications, and Ambulance Services. This Director also supervises the Medical Records relevant to Ambulance Services, the educational training for Security and Ambulance Services personnel, and the human resources for Security, Communications, and Ambulance Services personnel.

Required

Of the duties and services described above, all of which are supervised by one Director, which areas should be Responsibility Centers and which areas should be Support Centers? Draw them in a visual and indicate the reporting requirements.

Assignment Exercise 6–2: Responsibility Centers

Choose among the Physician's Practice in Mini-Case Study 2, the Clinic in Mini-Case Study 3, or Continuing Care Retirement Center in Mini-Case Study 1. Designate the Responsibility Centers and the Support Centers for the organization selected. Prepare a rationale for the structure you have designed.

CHAPTER 7

Example 7A: Fixed, Variable, and Semivariable Distinction

Review the chapter text for the distinction between fixed, variable, and semivariable costs. Pay particular attention to the accompanying Figures 7–1, 7–2, 7–3, 7–4, and 7–5.

Practice Exercise 7–I: Analyzing Mixed Costs

The Metropolis Health System has a system-wide training course for nurse aides. The course requires a packet of materials that MHS calls the *training pack*. Due to turnover and because the course is system-wide, there is a monthly demand for new packs. In addition the local community college also obtains the training packs used in their credit courses from MHS.

The Education Coordinator needs to know how much of the cost is fixed and how much of the cost is variable for these training packs. She decides to use the high-low method of computation.

Required

Using the monthly utilization information presented below, find the fixed and variable portion of costs through the high-low method.

Month	Number of Training Packs	Cost
January	1,000	$6,200
February	200	1,820
March	250	2,350
April	400	3,440
May	700	4,900
June	300	2,730
July	150	1,470
August	100	1,010
September	1,100	7,150
October	300	2,850
November	250	2,300
December	100	1,010

Assignment Exercise 7–1: Analyzing Mixed Costs

The Education Coordinator decides that the Community College packs may be unduly influencing the high-low computation. She decides to re-run the results omitting the Community College volume.

Required

1. Using the monthly utilization information presented below, and omitting the Community College training packs, find the fixed and variable portion of costs through

the high-low method. Note that the college only acquires packs in three months of the year: January, May, and September. These dates coincide with the start dates of their semesters and summer school.

2. The reason the Education Coordinator needs to know how much of the cost is fixed is because she is supposed to collect the appropriate variable cost from the Community College for their packs. For her purposes, which computation do you believe is better? Why?

Month	Total Number of Training Packs	Total Cost	Community College Number Packs	Community College Cost
January	1,000	$6,200	200	$1,240
February	200	1,820		
March	250	2,350		
April	400	3,440		
May	700	4,900	300	2,100
June	300	2,730		
July	150	1,470		
August	100	1,010		
September	1,100	7,150	300	1,950
October	300	2,850		
November	250	2,300		
December	100	1,010		

Example 7B: Contribution Margin

Computation of a contribution margin is simplified if the fixed and variable expense has already been determined. Examine Table 7–1, which contains Operating Room Fixed and Variable Costs. We can see that the total costs are $1,217,756. Of this amount, $600,822 is designated as variable cost and $616,934 is designated as fixed ($529,556 + $87,378 = $616,934). For purposes of our example, assume the Operating Room revenue amounts to $1,260,000. The contribution margin is computed as follows:

	Amount
Revenue	$1,260,000
Less Variable Cost	(600,822)
Contribution Margin	$659,178

Thus $659,178 is available to contribute to fixed costs and to profit. (In this example fixed costs amount to $616,934, so there is an amount left to contribute toward profit.)

Practice Exercise 7–II: Calculating the Contribution Margin

Greenside Clinic has revenue totaling $3,500,000. The clinic has costs totaling $3,450,000. Of this amount, 40 percent is variable cost and 60 percent is fixed cost.

Required

Compute the contribution margin for Greenside Clinic.

Assignment Exercise 7–2: Calculating the Contribution Margin

The Mental Health program for the Community Center has just completed its fiscal year end. The Program Director determines that his program has revenue for the year of $1,210,000. He believes his variable expense amounts to $205,000 and he knows his fixed expense amounts to $1,100,000.

Required

1. Compute the contribution margin for the Community Center Mental Health program.
2. What does the result tell you about the program?

Example 7C: Cost-Volume-Profit (CVP) Ratio and Profit-Volume (PV) Ratio

Closely review the examples of ratio calculations in the chapter text. Also note that examples are presented in visuals as well as text.

Practice Exercise 7–III: Calculating the PV Ratio

The Profit-Volume (PV) Ratio is also known as the Contribution Margin (CM) Ratio. Use the same assumptions for the Community Center Mental Health Program. In addition to the contribution margin figures already computed, now compute the PV Ratio (also known as CM Ratio).

Assignment Exercise 7–3: Calculating the PV Ratio and the CVP Ratio

Use the same assumptions for the Greenside Clinic. One more assumption will be added: the Clinic had 35,000 visits.

Required

1. In addition to the contribution margin figures already computed, now compute the PV Ratio (also known as CM Ratio).
2. Add another column to your worksheet and compute the clinic's per-visit revenue and costs.
3. Create a Cost-Volume-Profit chart. Refer to the chapter text along with Figure 7–6.

CHAPTER 8

Example 8A

Review the chapter text about annualizing positions. In particular review Exhibit 8–2, which contains the annualizing calculations.

Practice Exercise 8–I: FTEs to Annualize Staffing

The office manager for a physicians' group affiliated with Metropolis Health System is working on her budget for next year. She wants to annualize her staffing plan. To do so she needs to convert her staff's net paid days worked to a factor. Their office is open and staffed seven days a week, per their agreement with two managed care plans.

The office manager has the MHS work sheet, which shows 9 holidays, 7 sick days, 15 vacation days, and 3 education days, equaling 34 paid days per year not worked. The physicians' group allows 8 holidays, 5 sick days, and 1 education day. An employee must work one full year to earn 5 vacation days. An employee must have worked full time for three full years before earning 10 annual vacation days. Because the turnover is so high, nobody on staff has earned more than 5 vacation days.

Required

1. Compute Net Paid Days Worked for a full-time employee in the physicians' group.
2. Convert Net Paid Days Worked to a factor so the office manager can annualize her staffing plan.

Assignment Exercise 8–1: FTEs to Annualize Staffing

The Metropolis Health System managers are also working on their budgets for next year. Each manager must annualize his or her staffing plan, and thus must convert staff net paid days worked to a factor. Each manager has the MHS work sheet, which shows 9 holidays, 7 sick days, 15 vacation days, and 3 education days, equaling 34 paid days per year not worked.

The Laboratory is fully staffed seven days per week and the 34 paid days per year not worked is applicable for the lab. The Medical Records department is also fully staffed seven days per week. However, Medical Records is an outsourced department so the employee benefits are somewhat different. The Medical Records employees receive 9 holidays plus 21 personal leave days which can be used for any purpose.

Required

1. Compute Net Paid Days Worked for a full-time employee in the Laboratory and in Medical Records.
2. Convert Net Paid Days Worked to a factor for the Laboratory and for Medical Records so these MHS managers can annualize their staffing plans.

Example 8B

Review the chapter text about staffing requirements to fill a position. In particular review Exhibit 8–4, which contains (at the bottom of the exhibit) the staffing calculations. Remember this method uses a basic work week as the standard.

Practice Exercise 8–II: FTEs to Fill a Position

Metropolis Health System (MHS) uses a basic work week of 40 hours throughout the system. Thus one full-time employee works 40 hours per week. MHS also uses a standard 24-hour scheduling system of three 8-hour shifts. The Admissions manager needs to compute the staffing requirements to fill his departmental positions. He has more than one Admissions office staffed within the system. The West Admissions office typically has two Admissions officers on duty during the day shift, one Admissions officer on duty during the evening shift, and one Admissions officer on duty during the night shift. The day shift also has one clerical person on duty. Staffing is identical for all seven days of the week.

Required

1. Set up a staffing requirements worksheet, using the format in Exhibit 8–4.
2. Compute the number of FTEs required to fill the Admissions officer position and the clerical position at the West Admissions office.

Assignment Exercise 8–2: FTEs to Fill a Position

Metropolis Health System (MHS) uses a basic work week of 40 hours throughout the system. Thus one full-time employee works 40 hours per week. MHS also uses a standard 24-hour scheduling system of three 8-hour shifts. The Director of Nursing needs to compute the staffing requirements to fill the Operating Room positions. Since MHS is a trauma center the OR is staffed 24 hours a day, 7 days a week. At present, staffing is identical for all seven days of the week, although the Director of Nursing is questioning the efficiency of this method.

The Operating Room Department is staffed with two nursing supervisors on the day shift and one nursing supervisor apiece on the evening and night shifts. There are two technicians on the day shift, two technicians on the evening shift, and one technician on the night shift. There are three RNs on the day shift, two RNs on the evening shift, and one RN plus one LPN on the night shift. In addition there is one aide plus one clerical on the day shift only.

Required

1. Set up a staffing requirements worksheet, using the format in Exhibit 8–4.
2. Compute the number of FTEs required to fill the Operating Room staffing positions.

CHAPTER 9

Practice Exercise 9–I: Components of Balance Sheet and Statement of Net Income

Financial statements for Doctors Smith and Brown are provided below. Use the doctors' Balance Sheet, Statement of Revenue and Expenses, and Statement of Capital for this assignment.

Required

Identify the following doctors' Balance Sheet and Statement of Net Income components. List the name of each component and its amount(s) from the appropriate financial statement.

Current Liabilities
Total Assets
Income from Operations
Accumulated Depreciation
Total Operating Revenue
Current Portion of Long-Term Debt
Interest Income
Inventories

Assignment Exercise 9–1: Components of Balance Sheet and Statement of Net Income

Refer to the Metropolis Health System (MHS) Supplemental Information at the back of the Examples and Exercises section. Use the MHS comparative Balance Sheet, Statement of Revenue and Expenses, and Statement of Fund Balance for this assignment.

Required

Identify the following MHS Balance Sheet components. List the name of each component and its amount(s) from the appropriate MHS financial statement.

Current Liabilities
Total Assets
Income from Operations
Accumulated Depreciation
Total Operating Revenue
Current Portion of Long-Term Debt
Interest Income
Inventories

Doctors Smith and Brown
Statement of Net Income
for the Three Months Ended March 31, 20X7

Revenue		
Net patient service revenue	180,000	
Other revenue	-0-	
Total Operating Revenue		180,000
Expenses		
Nursing/PA salaries	16,650	
Clerical salaries	10,150	
Payroll taxes/employee benefits	4,800	
Medical supplies and drugs	15,000	
Professional fees	3,000	
Dues and publications	2,400	
Janitorial service	1,200	
Office supplies	1,500	
Repairs and maintenance	1,200	
Utilities and telephone	6,000	
Depreciation	30,000	
Interest	3,100	
Other	5,000	
Total Expenses		100,000
Income from Operations		80,000
Nonoperating Gains (Losses)		
Interest Income		-0-
Nonoperating Gains, Net		-0-
Net Income		80,000

Doctors Smith and Brown
Balance Sheet
March 31, 20X7

Assets

Current Assets

Cash and cash equivalents	25,000	
Patient accounts receivable	40,000	
Inventories—supplies and drugs	5,000	
Total Current Assets		70,000

Property, Plant and Equipment

Buildings and Improvements	500,000	
Equipment	800,000	
Total	1,300,000	
Less Accumulated Depreciation	(480,000)	
Net Depreciable Assets	820,000	
Land	100,000	
Property, Plant and Equipment, Net		920,000
Other Assets		10,000
Total Assets		1,000,000

Liabilities and Capital

Current Liabilities

Current maturities of long-term debt	10,000	
Accounts payable and accrued expenses	20,000	
Total Current Liabilities		30,000
Long-Term Debt	180,000	
Less Current Portion of Long-Term Debt	(10,000)	
Net Long-Term Debt		170,000
Total Liabilities		200,000
Capital		800,000
Total Liabilities and Capital		1,000,000

Doctors Smith and Brown
Statement of Changes in Capital
for the Three Months Ended March 31, 20X7

Beginning Balance	$720,000
Net Income	80,000
Ending Balance	$800,000

Example 9B: Depreciation Concept

Assume that MHS purchased equipment for $200,000 cash on April 1st (the first day of its fiscal year). This equipment has an expected life of 10 years. The salvage value is 10 percent of cost. No equipment was traded in on this purchase.

Straight-line depreciation is a method that charges an equal amount of depreciation for each year the asset is in service. In the case of this purchase, straight-line depreciation would amount to $18,000 per year for 10 years. This amount is computed as follows:

Step 1. Compute the cost net of salvage or trade-in value: 200,000 less 10 percent salvage value or 20,000 equals 180,000.

Step 2. Divide the resulting figure by the expected life (also known as estimated useful life): 180,000 divided by 10 equals 18,000 depreciation per year for 10 years.

Accelerated depreciation represents methods that are speeded up, or accelerated. In other words a greater amount of depreciation is taken earlier in the life of the asset. One example of accelerated depreciation is the double declining balance method. Unlike straight-line depreciation, trade-in or salvage value is not taken into account until the end of the depreciation schedule. This method uses *book value*, which is the net amount remaining when cumulative previous depreciation is deducted from the asset's cost. The computation is as follows:

Step 1. Compute the straight-line rate: 1 divided by 10 equals 10 percent.

Step 2. Now double the rate (as in *double declining method*): 10 percent times 2 equals 20 percent.

Step 3. Compute the first year's depreciation expense: 200,000 times 20 percent equals 40,000.

Step 4. Compute the carry-forward book value at the beginning of the second year: 200,000 book value beginning Year 1 less Year 1 depreciation of 40,000 equals book value at beginning of the second year of 160,000.

Step 5. Compute the second year's depreciation expense: 160,000 times 20 percent equals 32,000.

Step 6. Compute the carry-forward book value at the beginning of the third year: 160,000 book value beginning Year 2 less Year 2 depreciation of 32,000 equals book value at beginning of the third year of 128,000.
—Continue until the asset's salvage or trade-in value has been reached.
—Do not depreciate beyond the salvage or trade-in value.

Practice Exercise 9–II: Depreciation Concept

Assume that MHS purchased equipment for $600,000 cash on April 1st (the first day of its fiscal year). This equipment has an expected life of 10 years. The salvage value is 10 percent of cost. No equipment was traded in on this purchase.

Required

1. Compute the straight-line depreciation for this purchase.
2. Compute the double declining balance depreciation for this purchase.

Assignment Exercise 9–2: Depreciation Concept

Assume that MHS purchased two additional pieces of equipment on April 1st (the first day of its fiscal year), as follows:

(1) The laboratory equipment cost $300,000 and has an expected life of 5 years. The salvage value is 5 percent of cost. No equipment was traded in on this purchase.

(2) The radiology equipment cost $800,000 and has an expected life of 7 years. The salvage value is 10 percent of cost. No equipment was traded in on this purchase.

Required

For both pieces of equipment:

1. Compute the straight-line depreciation.
2. Compute the double declining balance depreciation.

CHAPTER 10

Example 10A

To better understand how the information for the numerator and the denominator of each calculation is obtained, Figure 10–1, Examples of Liquidity Ratio Calculations, illustrates the process. This figure takes the balance sheet and the statement of revenue and expense that were discussed in the preceding chapter and illustrates the source of each figure in the four liquidity ratios. The multiple computations in Days Cash on Hand and in Days Receivables are further broken out into a three-step process to better illustrate sources of information.

Practice Exercise 10–I: Liquidity Ratios

Two of the liquidity ratios are illustrated in this practice exercise. Refer to the Doctors Smith and Brown financial statements presented in preceding Chapter 9.

Required

1. Set up a worksheet for the current ratio and the quick ratio.
2. Compute the ratios for Doctors Smith and Brown.

Assignment Exercise 10–1: Liquidity Ratios

Refer to the Metropolis Health System (MHS) case study in Chapter 18.

Required

1. Set up a worksheet for the liquidity ratios.
2. Compute the four liquidity ratios using the Chapter 18 MHS financial statements.

Example 10B

To better understand how the information for the numerator and the denominator of each calculation is obtained, Figure 10–2, Examples of Solvency and Profitability Ratio Calculations, illustrates the process. This figure takes the balance sheet and the statement of revenue and expense that were discussed in the preceding chapter and illustrates the source of each figure in the two solvency ratios. Any multiple computations are further broken out to better explain sources of information.

Practice Exercise 10–II: Solvency Ratios

Refer to the Doctors Smith and Brown financial statements presented in preceding Chapter 9.

Required

1. Set up a worksheet for the solvency ratios.
2. Compute these ratios for Doctors Smith and Brown. To do so, you will need one additional piece of information that is not present on the doctors' statements: their maximum annual debt service is $22,200.

Assignment Exercise 10–2: Solvency Ratios

Refer to the Metropolis Health System (MHS) case study in Chapter 18.

Required

1. Set up a worksheet for the liquidity ratios.
2. Compute the solvency ratios using the Chapter 18 MHS financial statements.

Example 10C

To better understand how the information for the numerator and the denominator of each calculation is obtained, study Figure 10–2, Examples of Solvency and Profitability Ratio Calculations. This figure takes the balance sheet and the statement of revenue and expense that were discussed in the preceding chapter and illustrates the source of each figure in the two profitability ratios. Any multiple computations are further broken out to better explain sources of information.

Practice Exercise 10–III: Profitability Ratios

Refer to the Doctors Smith and Brown financial statements presented in preceding Chapter 9.

Required

1. Set up a worksheet for the profitability ratios.

2. Compute these ratios for Doctors Smith and Brown. All the necessary information is present on the doctors' statements.
    [Hint: "Operating Income (Loss)" is also known as "Income from Operations."]

Assignment Exercise 10–3: Profitability Ratios

Refer to the Metropolis Health System (MHS) case study in Chapter 18.

Required

1. Set up a worksheet for the liquidity ratios.
2. Compute the profitability ratios using the Chapter 18 MHS financial statements.

CHAPTER 11

Example 11A: Unadjusted Rate of Return

Assumptions:

- Average annual net income = $100,000
- Original investment amount = $1,000,000
- Unrecovered asset cost at the end of useful life (salvage value) = $100,000

Calculation using original investment amount:

$$\frac{\$\ 100,000}{\$1,000,000} = 10\% \text{ Unadjusted Rate of Return}$$

Calculation using average investment amount:

First Step: Compute average investment amount for total unrecovered asset cost.

At beginning of estimated useful life	=	$1,000,000
At end of estimated useful life	=	$ 100,000
	Sum	$1,100,000

Divided by 2 = $550,000 average investment amount

Second Step: Calculate unadjusted rate of return.

$$\frac{\$100,000}{\$550,000} = 18.2\% \text{ Unadjusted Rate of Return}$$

Practice Exercise 11–I: Unadjusted Rate of Return

Assumptions:

- Average annual net income = $100,000
- Original investment amount = $500,000
- Unrecovered asset cost at the end of useful life (salvage value) = $50,000

Required

1. Compute the Unadjusted Rate of Return using the original investment amount.
2. Compute the Unadjusted Rate of Return using the average investment method.

Assignment Exercise 11–1: Unadjusted Rate of Return

Metropolis Health Systems' Laboratory Director expects to purchase a new piece of equipment. The assumptions for the transaction are as follows:

- Average annual net income = $70,000
- Original investment amount = $410,000
- Unrecovered asset cost at the end of useful life (salvage value) = $41,000

Required

1. Compute the Unadjusted Rate of Return using the original investment amount.
2. Compute the Unadjusted Rate of Return using the average investment method.

Example 11B: Finding the Future Value (with a Compound Interest Table)

Betty Dylan is Director of Nurses at Metropolis Health System. Her oldest son will be entering college in five years. Today Betty is trying to figure what his college fund will amount to in five more years. (Hint: Compound interest means interest is not only earned on the principal, but also is earned on the previous interest earnings that have been left in the account. Interest is thus *compounded.*)

The college fund savings account presently has a balance of $9,000 and any interest earned over the next five years will be left in the account. Betty assumes the annual interest rate will be 6 percent. How much money will be in the account at the end of five more years?

Solution to Example

Step 1. Refer to the Compound Interest Table found in Appendix 11B at the back of this chapter. Reading across, or horizontally, find the 6 percent column. Reading down, or vertically, find Year 5. Trace across the Year 5 line item to the 6 percent column. The factor is 1.338.

Step 2. Multiply the current savings account balance of $9,000 times the factor of 1.338 to find the future value of $12,042. In five years at compound interest of 6 percent the college fund will have a balance of $12,042.

Practice Exercise 11–II: Finding the Future Value (with a Compound Interest Table)

Assume the college savings fund in the preceding example presently has a balance of $11,000 and any interest earned will be left in the account. Assume the annual interest rate will be 7 percent.

Required

Compute how much money will be in the account at the end of six more years. (Use the Future Value or Compound Interest Table found at the back of this chapter.)

Assignment Exercise 11–2: Finding the Future Value (with a Compound Interest Table)

John Whitten is one of the physicians on staff at Metropolis Health System. His practice is six years old. He has set up an office savings account to accumulate the funds to replace equipment in his practice. Today John is trying to figure what his equipment fund will amount to in four more years.

The equipment fund savings account presently has a balance of $63,500 and any interest earned over the next four years will be left in the account. John assumes the annual interest rate will be 5 percent. How much money will be in the account at the end of four more years?

Required

Compute how much money will be in the account at the end of four more years. (Use the Future Value or Compound Interest Table found at the back of this chapter.)

Example 11C: Finding the Present Value (with a Present Value Table)

Betty Dylan is taking an adult education night course in personal finance at the community college. The class is presently studying retirement planning. Each student is to estimate the amount of funds (in addition to pension plans and social security) they believe will be needed at retirement. Then they are to make a retirement plan.

Betty has estimated she would need $100,000 fifteen years from now. In order to complete her assignment she needs to know the present value of the $100,000. Betty further assumes an interest rate of 6 percent.

Solution to Example

Step 1. Refer to the Present Value Table found in Appendix 11-A at the back of this chapter. Reading across, or horizontally, find the 6 percent column. Reading down, or vertically, find Year 15. Trace across the Year 15 line item to the 6 percent column. The factor is 0.4173.

Step 2. Multiply $100,000 times the factor of 0.4173 to find the present value of $41,730.

Practice Exercise 11–III: Finding the Present Value (with a Present Value Table)

Betty isn't finished with her assignment. Now she wants to find the present value of $150,000 accumulated fifteen years from now. She further assumes a better interest rate of 7 percent.

Required

Compute the present value of $150,000 accumulated fifteen years from now. Assume an interest rate of 7 percent. (Use the Present Value Table found at the back of this chapter.)

Assignment Exercise 11–3: Finding the Present Value (with a Present Value Table)

Part 1—Dr. John Whitten is still figuring on his equipment fund. According to his calculations he needs $250,000 to be accumulated six years from now. John is now trying to find the present value of the $250,000. He continues to assume an interest rate of 5 percent.

Required

Compute the present value of $250,000 accumulated fifteen years from now. Assume an interest rate of 5 percent. (Use the Present Value Table found at the back of this chapter.)

   Part 2—John doesn't like the answer he gets. What, he thinks, if he can raise the interest rate to 7 percent? How much difference would that make?

Required

Compute the present value of $250,000 accumulated fifteen years from now assuming an interest rate of 7 percent. Compare the difference between this amount and the present value at 5 percent.

Example 11D: Internal Rate of Return

Review the chapter text to follow the steps set out to compute internal rate of return.

Practice Exercise 11–IV: Internal Rate of Return

Metropolis Health System (MHS) is considering purchasing a tractor to mow the grounds. It would cost $16,950 and have a 10-year useful life. It will have zero salvage value at the end of 10 years. The head of the MHS grounds crew estimates it would save $3,000 per year. He figures this savings because just one of the present maintenance crew would be driving the tractor, replacing the labor of several men now using small household-type lawn mowers. Compute the internal rate of return for this proposed acquisition.

Assignment Exercise 11–4: Computing an Internal Rate of Return

Dr. Whitten has decided to purchase equipment that has a cost of $60,000 and will produce a pretax net cash inflow of $30,000 per year over its estimated useful life of six years. The equipment will have no salvage value and will be depreciated by the straight-line method. The tax rate is 50 percent. Determine Dr. Whitten's approximate after-tax internal rate of return.

Example 11E: Payback Period

Review the chapter text and follow the Doctor Green detailed example of payback period computation.

Practice Exercise 11–V: Payback

The MHS Chief Financial Officer is considering a request by the Emergency Room Department for purchase of new equipment. It will cost $500,000. There is no trade-in. Its useful life would be 10 years. This type of machine is new to the department but it is estimated that it will result in $84,000 annual revenue and operating costs would be one-quarter of that amount. The CFO wants to find the payback period for this piece of equipment.

Assignment Exercise 11–5: Payback Period

The MHS Chief Financial Officer is considering alternate proposals for the hospital radiology department. The Director of Radiology has suggested purchasing one of two pieces of equipment. Machine A costs $15,000 and Machine B costs $12,000. Both machines are estimated to reduce radiology operating costs by $5,000 per year.

Required

Which machine should be purchased? Make your payback calculations to provide the answer.

CHAPTER 12

Example 12A: Common Sizing

Common sizing converts numbers to percentages so that comparative analysis can be performed. Reread the chapter text about common sizing and examine the percentages shown in Table 12–1.

Practice Exercise 12–I: Common Sizing

The worksheet below shows the assets of two hospitals.

Required

Perform common sizing for the assets of the two hospitals.

	Same Year for Both Hospitals	
	Hospital A	Hospital B
Current Assets	$ 2,000,000	$ 8,000,000
Property, Plant & Equipment	7,500,000	30,000,000
Other Assets	500,000	2,000,000
Total Assets	$10,000,000	$40,000,000

Assignment Exercise 12–1: Common Sizing

Refer to the Metropolis Health System (MHS) comparative financial statements at the back of the Examples and Exercises section.

Required

Common size the MHS Statement of Revenue and Expenses.

Example 12B: Trend Analysis

Trend analysis allows comparison of figures over time. Reread the chapter text about trend analysis and examine the *difference* columns shown in Table 12–3.

Practice Exercise 12–II: Trend Analysis

The worksheet below shows the assets of Hospital A over two years.

Required

Perform trend analysis for the assets of Hospital A.

	Hospital A	
	Year 1	*Year 2*
Current Assets	$1,600,000	$ 2,000,000
Property, Plant & Equipment	6,000,000	7,500,000
Other Assets	400,000	500,000
Total Assets	$8,000,000	$10,000,000

Assignment Exercise 12–2: Trend Analysis

Refer to the Metropolis Health System (MHS) comparative financial statements at the back of the Examples and Exercises section.

Required

Perform trend analysis on the MHS Statement of Revenue and Expenses.

Assignment Exercise 12–3: Benchmarking

Review the chapter text about benchmarking.

Required

1. Select either the MHS case study in Chapter 18 or one of the organizations represented by a mini-case study in Chapters 19 or 20.
2. Prepare a list of measures that could be benchmarked for this organization. Comment on why these items are important for benchmarking purposes.
3. Find another example of benchmarking for a health care organization. The example

can be an organization report or it can be taken from a published source such as a journal article.

Assignment Exercise 12–4: Pareto Rule

Review the chapter text about the Pareto rule and examine Figure 12–3. Note that the text says Pareto diagrams are often drawn to reflect *before* and *after* results.

Assume that Figure 12–3 is the *before* diagram for the Billing Department. Further assume that the *after* results are as follows:

Activity	Activity Code	Number
Process Denied Bills	PDB	12
Review with Supervisor	RWS	10
Locate Documentation	LD	6
Copy Documentation	CD	5
		33

Required

1. Redo the Pareto diagram with the *after* results. (Use Figure 12–3 as a guide.)
2. Comment on the *before* and *after* results for the Billing Department.

CHAPTER 13

Example 13A: Budgeting

A static budget is based on a single level of operations, which is never adjusted. Therefore the static budgeted expense amounts will not change even though actual volume does change during the year.

The computation of a static budget variance only requires one calculation, as follows:

$$\text{Actual results} \quad \text{minus} \quad \text{Static budget amount} \quad \text{equals} \quad \text{Static budget variance}$$

We can set up the example in the chapter text in this format as follows.

Use patient days as an example of level of volume, or output. Assume that the budget anticipated 40,000 patient days this year at an average of $600 revenue per day, or $2,400,000. Further assume that expenses were budgeted at $560 per patient day, or $22,400,000. The budget would look like this:

	As Budgeted
Revenue	$24,000,000
Expenses	22,400,000
Excess of Revenue over Expenses	$ 1,600,000

Now assume that only 36,000, or 90 percent, of the patient days are going to actually be achieved for the year. The average revenue of $600 per day will be achieved for these 36,000 days (thus 36,000 times 600 equals 21,600,000). Further assume that, despite the best efforts of the Chief Financial Officer, the expenses will amount to $22,000,000. The actual results would look like this:

	Actual
Revenue	$21,600,000
Expenses	22,000,000
Excess of Expenses over Revenue	$ (400,000)

The budgeted revenue and expenses still reflect the original expectation of 40,000 patient days; the budget report would look like this:

	Actual	*Budget*	*Static Budget Variance*
Revenue	$21,600,000	$24,000,000	$(2,400,000)
Expenses	22,000,000	22,400,000	(400,000)
Excess of Expenses over Revenue	$ (400,000)	$ 1,600,000	$(2,000,000)

Note: The negative actual result of (400,000) combined with the positive budget expectation of 1,600,000 amounts to the negative net variance of (2,000,000).

This example has shown a static budget, geared toward only one level of activity and remaining constant or static.

Practice Exercise 13–I: Budgeting

Budget assumptions for this exercise include both inpatient and outpatient revenue and expense. Assumptions are as follows:
As to the initial budget:

- The budget anticipated 30,000 inpatient days this year at an average of $650 revenue per day.
- Inpatient expenses were budgeted at $600 per patient day.
- The budget anticipated 10,000 outpatient visits this year at an average of $400 revenue per visit.
- Outpatient expenses were budgeted at $380 per visit.

As to the actual results:

- Assume that only 27,000, or 90 percent, of the inpatient days are going to actually be achieved for the year.
- The average revenue of $650 per day will be achieved for these 270,000 inpatient days.
- The outpatient visits will actually amount to 110 percent, or 11,000 for the year.
- The average revenue of $400 per visit will be achieved for these 11,000 visits.
- Further assume that, due to the heroic efforts of the Chief Financial Officer, the actual inpatient expenses will amount to $11,600,000 and the actual outpatient expenses will amount to $4,000,000.

Required

1. Set up three worksheets that follow the format of those in Example 13A. However, in each of your worksheets make two lines for Revenue; label one as *Revenue-Inpatient* and the other *Revenue-Outpatient*. Add a *Revenue Subtotal* line. Likewise, make two lines for *Expense*; label one as *Expense-Inpatient* and the other *Expense-Outpatient*. Add an *Expense Subtotal* line.
2. Using the new assumptions, complete the first worksheet for "As Budgeted."
3. Using the new assumptions, complete the second worksheet for "Actual."
4. Using the new assumptions, complete the third worksheet for "Static Budget Variance."

Assignment Exercise 13–1: Budgeting

Select an organization; either Metropolis Health System from the Chapter 18 Case Study or one of the organizations presented in the Mini-Case Studies in Chapters 19–21.

Required

1. Using the organization selected, create a budget for the next fiscal year. Set out the details of all assumptions you needed in order to build this budget.
2. Use the Checklist for Building a Budget (Exhibit 13–2) and critique your own budget.

Assignment Exercise 13–2: Budgeting

Find an existing budget from a published source. Detail should be extensive enough to present a challenge.

Required

1. Using the existing budget, create a new budget for the next fiscal year. Set out the details of all assumptions you needed in order to build this budget.
2. Use the Checklist for Building a Budget (Exhibit 13–2) and critique your own effort.
3. Use the Checklist for Reviewing a Budget (Exhibit 13–1) and critique the existing budget.

Example 13B: Variance Analysis

Our variance analysis example and practice exercise use the flexible budget approach. A flexible budget is one that is created using budgeted revenue and/or budgeted cost amounts. A flexible budget is adjusted, or flexed, to the actual level of output achieved (or perhaps expected to be achieved) during the budget period. A flexible budget thus looks toward a range of activity or volume (versus only one level in the static budget).

Examples of how the variance analysis works are contained in Figure 13–1 (the elements), in Figure 13–2 (the composition), and in Figures 13–3 and 13–4 (the calculation). Study these examples before undertaking the Practice Exercise.

Practice Exercise 13–II: Variance Analysis

Exhibit 13–4 presents a Summary Variance Report for the nursing activity center of St. Joseph Hospital for the month of September. For our practice exercise we will duplicate this report for the month of March.

Assumptions are as follows:

- Actual Activity Level is 687,000.
- Budgeted Activity Level is 650,000.
- Actual Cost per RVU is $4.70.
- Budgeted Cost per RVU is $5.00.
- Actual Overhead Costs are $3,228,900.
- Budgeted Overhead Costs are $3,250,000.

Required

1. Set up a worksheet for the month of March like that shown in Exhibit 13–4 for the month of September.
2. Insert the March Input Data (per assumptions given above) on the worksheet.
3. Complete the "Actual Costs," "Flexible Budget," and "Budgeted Costs" sections at the top of the worksheet.
4. Compute the Price Variance and the Quantity Variance in the middle of the worksheet.
5. Indicate whether the Price and the Quantity Variances are favorable or unfavorable for March.

Optional

Can you compute how the $3,228,900 actual overhead costs and the $3,250,000 budgeted overhead costs were calculated?

Assignment Exercise 13–3: Variance Analysis

Greenview Hospital operated at 120 percent of normal capacity in two of its departments during the year. It operated 120 percent times 20,000 normal capacity direct labor nursing hours in routine services and it operated 120 percent times 20,000 normal capacity equipment hours in the laboratory. The lab allocates overhead by measuring minutes and hours the equipment is used; thus *equipment hours*.

Assumptions:

For Routine Services Nursing:
- 20,000 hours × 120% = 24,000 direct labor nursing hours.
- Budgeted Overhead at 24,000 hours = $42,000 fixed plus $6,000 variable = $48,000 total.
- Actual Overhead at 24,000 hours = $42,000 fixed plus $7,000 variable = $49,000 total.
- Applied Overhead for 24,000 hours at $2.35 @ = $56,400.

For Laboratory:
- 20,000 hours × 120% = 24,000 equipment hours.
- Budgeted Overhead at 24,000 hours = $59,600 fixed plus $11,400 variable = $71,000 total.
- Actual Overhead at 24,000 hours = $59,600 fixed plus $11,600 variable = $71,200 total.
- Applied Overhead for 24,000 hours at $3.455 @ = $82,920.

Required

1. Set up a worksheet for Applied Overhead Costs and Volume Variance with a column for Routine Services Nursing and a second column for Laboratory.
2. Set up a worksheet for Actual Overhead Costs and Budget Variance with a column for Routine Services Nursing and a second column for Laboratory.
3. Set up a worksheet for Volume Variance and Budget Variance totaling Net Variance with a column for Routine Services Nursing and a second column for Laboratory.
4. Insert input data from Assumptions.
5. Complete computations for all three worksheets.

CHAPTER 14

Example 14A: Description of Capital Expenditure Proposals Scoring System

Worthwhile Hospital has a total capital expenditure budget for next year of five million dollars. Of this amount, three million is already committed as spending for capital assets that have already been acquired and are in place. The remaining two million dollars is available for new assets and for new projects or programs.

Worthwhile Hospital typically divides the available capital expenditure funds into monies available for inpatient purposes and monies available for outpatient purposes. This year the split is proposed to be 50-50.

The hospital's CFO is also proposing that a scoring system be used to evaluate this year's proposals. She has set up a scoring system that allows a maximum of five points. Thus the low is a score of one point and the high is a score of five points.

In addition to the points earned by a funding proposal, the CFO will allow one "bonus point" for upgrading existing equipment and one "bonus point" for funding expansion of existing programs.

Practice Exercise 14–I: Capital Expenditure Proposals

Jody Smith, the Director who supervises the Intensive Care Units, wants to secure as much of the one million dollars available for inpatient purposes as is possible for the ICU. At the same time Ted Jones, the Director who supervises the Surgery Unit, also wants to secure as much of the one million dollars available for inpatient purposes as is possible for his Surgery Unit.

Given the CFO's new scoring system, how should Jody go about choosing exactly what to request?

Assignment Exercise 14–1: Capital Expenditure Proposals

Ted Jones, the Surgery Unit Director, is about to choose his strategy for creating a capital expenditure funding proposal for the coming year. Ted's unit needs more room. The Surgery Unit is running at over 90% capacity. In addition, a prominent cardiology surgeon on staff at the hospital wants to create a new cardiac surgery program that would require extensive funding for more space and for new state-of-the-art equipment. The surgeon has been campaigning with the hospital board members.

Required

What should Ted decide to ask for? How should he go about crafting a strategy to justify his request, given the hospital's new scoring system?

CHAPTER 15

Example 15A: Loan Amortization

This example illustrates the initial monthly payments of a loan with a principal balance of 50,000, an interest rate of ten percent, and a payment period of three years or thirty-six months
Loan Amortization Schedule
Principal borrowed: 50,000
Total payments: 36
Annual interest rate 10.00% (monthly rate = 0.8333%)

Payment #	Total Payment	Principal Portion of Payment	Interest Expense Portion of Payment	Remaining Principal Balance
			Beginning balance =	50,000.00
1	1,613.36	1,196.69	416.67	48,403.31
2	1,613.36	1,206.67	406.69	47,596.64
3	1,613.36	1,216.72	396.64	46,379.92
4	1,613.36	1,226.86	386.50	45,153.06
5	1,613.36	1,237.08	376.28	43,915.98
6	1,613.36	1,247.39	365.97	42,668.58

Practice Exercise 15–I: Loan Amortization

This exercise illustrates a different principal amount than Example 15A, but computed at the same monthly interest rate and the same number of payments.

Required

Compute the first six months of a loan amortization schedule with a principal balance of 60,000, an interest rate of ten percent, and a payment period of three years or thirty-six months.

Loan Amortization Schedule
Principal borrowed: 60,000
Total payments: 36
Annual interest rate 10.00% (monthly rate = 0.8333%)

Payment #	Total Payment	Principal Portion of Payment	Interest Expense Portion of Payment	Remaining Principal Balance
			Beginning balance =	60,000.00
1				
2				
3				
4				
5				
6				

Assignment Exercise 15–1: Financial Statement Capital Structures

Required

Find three different financial statements that have varying capital structures. Write a paragraph about each that explains the debt-equity relationship and that computes the percent of debt and the percent of equity represented.

Also note whether the percent of annual interest on debt is revealed in the notes to the financial statements. If so, do you believe the interest rate is fair and equitable? Why?

CHAPTER 16

Example 16A: Depreciation

This example shows straight line depreciation computed at a five-year useful life with no salvage value. Straight line depreciation is the method commonly used for financing projections and funding proposals.

Depreciation Expense Computation: Straight line
5-year useful life; no salvage value

Year #	*Annual* *Depreciation*	*Remaining* *Balance*
Beginning Balance =		60,000
1	12,000	48,000
2	12,000	36,000
3	12,000	24,000
4	12,000	12,000
5	12,000	-0-

Example 16B: Depreciation

This example shows straight line depreciation computed at a five-year useful life with a remaining salvage value of $10,000. Note the difference in annual depreciation between 16A and 16B.

Depreciation Expense Computation: Straightline
5-year useful life; $10,000 salvage value

Year #	*Annual* *Depreciation*	*Remaining* *Balance*
Beginning Balance =		60,000
1	10,000	50,000
2	10,000	40,000
3	10,000	30,000
4	10,000	20,000
5	10,000	10,000

Example 16C: Depreciation

This example shows double declining depreciation computed at a five-year useful life with no salvage value. As is often the case with a five-year life, the double declining method is used for the first three years and the straight line method is used for the remaining two years. The double declining method first computes what the straight-line percentage would be. In this case 100 percent divided by five years equals 20 percent. The 20 percent is then doubled. In this case 20 percent times 2 equals 40 percent. Then the 40 percent is multiplied times the remaining balance to be depreciated. Thus 60,000 times 40 percent for year one equals 24,000 depreciation, with a remaining balance of 36,000. Then 36,000 times 40 percent for year two equals 14,400 depreciation, and 36,000 minus 14,400 equals 21,600 remaining balance, and so on.

Now note the difference in annual depreciation between 16A, using straight-line for all five years, and 16C, using the combined double declining and straight line methods.

Depreciation Expense Computation: Double Declining Balance

5-year useful life; $10,000 salvage value

Year #	Annual Depreciation	Remaining Balance
Beginning Balance =		60,000
1	24,000 *	36,000
2	14,400 *	21,600
3	8,640 *	12,960
4	6,480 **	6,480
5	6,480 **	6,480

* = double declining balance depreciation
** = straight-line depreciation for remaining two years (12,960 divided by 2=6,480/yr)

Practice Exercise 16–I: Depreciation

Compute the straight line depreciation for equipment with a cost of $50,000, a 5-year useful life, and a $5,000 salvage value.

Assignment Exercise 16–1: Depreciation

Set up a purchase scenario of your own and compute the depreciation with and without salvage value.

Practice Exercise 16–II: Cost of Leasing

A cost of leasing table is reproduced below.

Required

Using the appropriate table from the Chapter 11 Appendices, record the present value factor at 6% for each year and compute the present value cost of leasing.

Cost of Leasing: Suburban Clinic—Comparative Present Value

Not-For-Profit Cost of Leasing:	Year 0	Year 1	Year 2	Year 3	Year 4	Year 5
Net Cash Flow	(11,000)	(11,000)	(11,000)	(11,000)	(11,000)	—
Present value factor (at 6%)						
Present value answer =						
Present value cost of leasing =						

Assignment Exercise 16–2: Cost of Owning and Cost of Leasing

Cost of owning and cost of leasing tables are reproduced below.

Required

Using the appropriate table from the Chapter 11 Appendices, record the present value factor at 10% for each year and compute the present value cost of owning and the present value of leasing. Which alternative is more desirable at this interest rate? Do you think your answer would change if the interest rate was six percent instead of ten percent?

Cost of Owning: Anywhere Clinic—Comparative Present Value

For-Profit Cost of Owning:	Year 0	Year 1	Year 2	Year 3	Year 4	Year 5
Net Cash Flow	(48,750)	2,500	2,500	2,500	2,500	5,000
Present value factor						
Present value answers =						
Present value cost of owning =						

Cost of Leasing: Anywhere Clinic—Comparative Present Value

Line #	*For-Profit Cost of Leasing:*	Year 0	Year 1	Year 2	Year 3	Year 4	Year 5
19	Net Cash Flow	(8,250)	(8,250)	(8,250)	(8,250)	(8,250)	—
20	Present value factor						
21	Present value answers =						
22	**Present value cost of leasing =**						

CHAPTER 17

Example 17A: Assumptions

Types of assumptions required for the financial portion of a business plan typically include answers to the following questions:

Example of Typical Income Statement Assumption Information Requirements:

- What types of revenue?
- How many services will be offered to produce the revenue? (by month)
- How much labor will be required? (FTEs)
- What will the labor cost?
- How many and what type of supplies, drugs and/or devices will be required to offer the service?
- What will the supplies, drugs and/or devices cost?
- How much space will be required?
- What will the required space occupancy cost?
- Is special equipment required?
- If so, how much will it cost?
- Is staff training required to use the special equipment?
- If so, how much time is required, and what will it cost?

Practice Exercise 17–I: Assumptions

Refer to the proposal to add a retail pharmacy mini-case study in Chapter 19.

Required

Identify how many of the assumption items listed in the example above can be found in the retail pharmacy proposal worksheets.

Assignment Exercise 17–1: Business Plan

Refer to the proposal to add a retail pharmacy mini-case study in Chapter 19.

Required

Build a Business Plan for this proposal. Prepare the service description using your consumer knowledge of a retail pharmacy (if necessary). Of course this retail pharmacy will be located within the hospital, but its purpose is to dispense prescriptions to carry off-site and use at home. Thus it operates pretty much like the neighborhood retail pharmacy that you use yourself.

   Use the information provided in Chapter 19 to prepare the financial section of the Business Plan. Use your imagination to create the marketing segment and the organization segment.

SUPPLEMENTAL MATERIALS

Present Value of an Annuity of $1

Periods	2%	4%	6%	8%	10%	12%	14%	16%	18%	20%	Periods
1	.980	.962	.943	.926	.909	.893	.877	.862	.848	.833	1
2	1.942	1.886	1.833	1.783	1.736	1.690	1.647	1.605	1.566	1.528	2
3	2.884	2.775	2.673	2.577	2.487	2.402	2.322	2.246	2.174	2.107	3
4	3.808	3.630	3.465	3.312	3.170	3.037	2.914	2.798	2.690	2.589	4
5	4.713	4.452	4.212	3.993	3.791	3.605	3.433	3.274	3.127	2.991	5
6	5.601	5.242	4.917	4.623	4.355	4.111	3.889	3.685	3.498	3.326	6
7	6.472	6.002	5.582	5.206	4.868	4.564	4.288	4.039	3.812	3.605	7
8	7.325	6.733	6.210	5.747	5.335	4.968	4.639	4.344	4.078	3.837	8
9	8.162	7.435	6.802	6.247	5.759	5.328	4.946	4.607	4.303	4.031	9
10	8.983	8.111	7.360	6.710	6.145	5.650	5.216	4.833	4.494	4.193	10
15	12.849	11.118	9.712	8.560	7.606	6.811	6.142	5.576	5.092	4.676	15
20	16.351	13.590	11.470	9.818	8.514	7.469	6.623	5.929	5.353	4.870	20
25	19.523	15.622	12.783	10.675	9.077	7.843	6.873	6.097	5.467	4.948	25

Metropolis Health System
Balance Sheet
March 31, 20X8 and 20X7

Assets

	20X8	20X7
Current Assets		
Cash and cash equivalents	1,150,000	400,000
Assets whose use is limited	825,000	825,000
Patient accounts receivable	8,700,000	8,950,000
Less allowance for bad debts	(1,300,000)	(1,300,000)
Other receivables	150,000	100,000
Inventories of supplies	900,000	850,000
Prepaid expenses	200,000	150,000
Total Current Assets	10,625,000	9,975,000
Assets Whose Use is Limited		
Corporate funded depreciation	1,950,000	1,800,000
Under bond indenture agreements—		
held by trustee	1,425,000	1,475,000
Total Assets Whose Use is Limited	3,375,000	3,275,000
Less Current Portion	(825,000)	(825,000)
Net Assets Whose Use is Limited	2,550,000	2,450,000
Property, Plant and Equipment, Net	19,300,000	19,200,000
Other Assets	325,000	375,000
Total Assets	32,800,000	32,000,000

Metropolis Health System
Balance Sheet
March 31, 20X8 and 20X7

Liabilities and Fund Balance

Current Liabilities

Current maturities of long-term debt	525,000	500,000
Accounts payable and accrued expenses	4,900,000	5,300,000
Bond interest payable	300,000	325,000
Reimbursement settlement payable	100,000	175,000
Total Current Liabilities	5,825,000	6,300,000
Long-Term Debt	6,000,000	6,500,000
Less Current Portion of Long-Term Debt	(525,000)	(500,000)
Net Long-Term Debt	5,475,000	6,000,000
Total Liabilities	11,300,000	12,300,000
Fund Balances		
General Fund	21,500,000	19,700,000
Total Fund Balances	21,500,000	19,700,000
Total Liabilities and Fund Balances	32,800,000	32,000,000

Metropolis Health System
Statement of Revenue and Expenses
for the Years Ended March 31, 20X8 and 20X7

Revenue			
Net patient service revenue	34,000,000		33,600,000
Other revenue	1,100,000		1,000,000
Total Operating Revenue		35,100,000	34,600,000
Expenses			
Nursing services	5,025,000		5,450,000
Other professional services	13,100,000		12,950,000
General services	3,200,000		3,220,000
Support services	8,300,000		8,340,000
Depreciation	1,900,000		1,800,000
Amortization	50,000		50,000
Interest	325,000		350,000
Provision for doubtful accounts	1,500,000		1,600,000
Total Expenses		33,400,000	33,760,000
Income from Operations		1,700,000	840,000
Nonoperating Gains (Losses)			
Unrestricted gifts and memorials	20,000		70,000
Interest income	80,000		40,000
Nonoperating Gains, Net		100,000	110,000
Revenue and Gains in Excess of Expenses and Losses		1,800,000	950,000

Metropolis Health System
Statement of Changes in Fund Balance
for the Years Ended March 31, 20X8 and 20X7

General Fund Balance April 1st	$19,700,000	$18,750,000
Revenue and Gains in Excess of Expenses and Losses	1,800,000	950,000
General Fund Balance March 31st	$21,500,000	$19,700,000

Metropolis Health System
Schedule of Property, Plant, and Equipment
for the Years Ended March 31, 20X8 and 20X7

Buildings and Improvements	14,700,000	14,000,000
Land Improvements	1,100,000	1,100,000
Equipment	28,900,000	27,600,000
Total	44,700,000	42,700,000
Less Accumulated Depreciation	(26,100,000)	(24,200,000)
Net Depreciable Assets	18,600,000	18,500,000
Land	480,000	480,000
Construction in Progress	220,000	220,000
Net Property, Plant, and Equipment	19,300,000	19,200,000

Metropolis Health System
Schedule of Patient Revenue
For the Years Ended March 31, 20X8 and 20X7

Patient Services Revenue		
Routine revenue	9,850,000	9,750,000
Laboratory	7,375,000	7,300,000
Radiology and CT scanner	5,825,000	5,760,000
OB–nursery	450,000	445,000
Pharmacy	3,175,000	3,140,000
Emergency service	2,200,000	2,180,000
Medical and surgical supply and IV	5,050,000	5,000,000
Operating rooms	5,250,000	5,200,000
Anesthesiology	1,600,000	1,580,000
Respiratory therapy	900,000	890,000
Physical therapy	1,475,000	1,460,000
EKG and EEG	1,050,000	1,040,000
Ambulance services	900,000	890,000
Oxygen	575,000	570,000
Home health and hospice	1,675,000	1,660,000
Substance abuse	375,000	370,000
Other	775,000	765,000
Subtotal	48,500,000	48,000,000
Less: Allowances and Charity Care	14,500,000	14,400,000
Net Patient Service Revenue	34,000,000	33,600,000

Metropolis Health System
Schedule of Operating Expenses
for the Years Ended March 31, 20X8 and 20X7

Nursing Services

Routine Medical-Surgical	3,880,000	4,200,000
Operating Room	300,000	325,000
Intensive Care Units	395,000	430,000
OB–Nursery	150,000	165,000
Other	300,000	330,000
Total	5,025,000	5,450,000

Other Professional Services

Laboratory	2,375,000	2,350,000
Radiology and CT Scanner	1,700,000	1,680,000
Pharmacy	1,375,000	1,360,000
Emergency Service	950,000	930,000
Medical and Surgical Supply	1,800,000	1,780,000
Operating Rooms and Anesthesia	1,525,000	1,515,000
Respiratory Therapy	525,000	530,000
Physical Therapy	700,000	695,000
EKG and EEG	185,000	180,000
Ambulance Services	80,000	80,000
Substance Abuse	460,000	450,000
Home Health and Hospice	1,295,000	1,280,000
Other	130,000	120,000
Total	13,100,000	12,950,000

General Services

Dietary	1,055,000	1,060,000
Maintenance	1,000,000	1,010,000
Laundry	295,000	300,000
Housekeeping	470,000	475,000
Security	50,000	50,000
Medical Records	330,000	325,000
Total	3,200,000	3,220,000

Support Services

General	4,600,000	4,540,000
Insurance	240,000	235,000
Payroll Taxes	1,130,000	1,180,000
Employee Welfare	1,900,000	1,950,000
Other	430,000	435,000
Total	8,300,000	8,340,000

Depreciation	1,900,000	1,800,000
Amortization	50,000	50,000
Interest Expense	325,000	350,000
Provision for Doubtful Accounts	1,500,000	1,600,000
Total Operating Expenses	33,400,000	33,760,000

EXCERPTS FROM METROPOLITAN HEALTH SYSTEM NOTES TO FINANCIAL STATEMENTS

Note 1—Nature of Operations and Summary of Significant Accounting Policies

General

Metropolitan Hospital System (Hospital) currently operates as a general acute care hospital. The Hospital is a municipal corporation and body politic created under the Hospital District laws of the State.

Cash and Cash Equivalents

For purposes of reporting cash flows, the Hospital considers all liquid investments with an original maturity of three months or less to be cash equivalents.

Inventory

Inventory consists of supplies used for patients and is stated at the lower of cost or market. Cost is determined on the basis of most recent purchase price.

Investments

Investments, consisting primarily of debt securities, are carried at market value. Realized and unrealized gains and losses are reflected in the statement of revenue and expenses. Investment income from general fund investments is reported as nonoperating gains.

Income Taxes

As a municipal corporation of the State, the Hospital is exempt from Federal and State income taxes under Section 115 of the Internal Revenue Code.

Property, Plant, and Equipment

Expenditures for property, plant, and equipment and items that substantially increase the useful lives of existing assets are capitalized at cost. The Hospital provides for depreciation on the straight-line method at rates designed to depreciate the costs of assets over estimated useful lives as follows:

	Years
Equipment	5 to 20
Land Improvements	20 to 25
Buildings and Improvements	40

Funded Depreciation

The Hospital's Board of Directors has adopted the policy of designating certain funds that are to be used to fund depreciation for the purpose of improvement, replacement, or expansion of plant assets.

Unamortized Debt Issue Costs

Revenue bond issue costs have been deferred and are being amortized.

Revenue and Gains in Excess of Expenses and Losses

The statement of revenue and expenses includes Revenue and Gains in Excess of Expenses and Losses. Changes in unrestricted net assets that are excluded from excess of revenue over expenses, consistent with industry practice, would include such items as contributions of long-lived assets (including assets acquired using contributions that by donor restriction were to be used for the purposes of acquiring such assets) and extraordinary gains and losses. Such items are not present on the current financial statements.

Net Patient Service Revenue

Net patient service revenue is reported at the estimated net realizable amounts from patients, third-party payers, and others for services rendered, including estimated retroactive adjustments under reimbursement agreements with third-party payers. Retroactive adjustments are accrued on an estimated basis in the period the related services are rendered and adjusted in future periods as final settlements are determined.

Contractual Agreements with Third-Party Payers

The Hospital has contractual agreements with third-party payers, primarily the Medicare and Medicaid programs. The Medicare program reimburses the Hospital for inpatient services under the Prospective Payment System, which provides for payment at predetermined amounts based on the discharge diagnosis. The contractual agreement with the Medicaid program provides for reimbursement based upon rates established by the State, subject to State appropriations. The difference between established customary charge rates and reimbursement is accounted for as a contractual allowance.

Gifts and Bequests

Unrestricted gifts and bequests are recorded on the accrual basis as nonoperating gains.

Donated Services

No amounts have been reflected in the financial statements for donated services. The Hospital pays for most services requiring specific expertise. However, many individuals volunteer their time and perform a variety of tasks that assists the Hospital with specific assistance programs and various committee assignments.

Note 2—Cash and Investments

Statutes require that all deposits of the Hospital be secured by federal depository insurance or be fully collateralized by the banking institution in authorized investments. Authorized investments include those guaranteed by the full faith and credit of the United States of America as to principal and interest; or in bonds, notes, debentures, or other similar obligations of the United States of America or its agencies; in interest-bearing savings accounts, interest-bearing certificates of deposit; or in certain money market mutual funds.

At March 31, 20X8, the carrying amount and bank balance of the Hospital's deposits with financial institutions were $190,000 and $227,000, respectively. The difference between the carrying amount and the bank balance primarily represents checks outstanding at March 31, 20X8. All deposits are fully insured by the Federal Deposit Insurance Corporation or collateralized with securities held in the Hospital's name by the Hospital agent.

	Carrying Amount	
	20X8	*20X7*
U.S. Government Securities or		
U.S. Government Agency Securities	4,325,000	3,575,000
Total Investments	4,325,000	3,575,000
Petty Cash	3,000	3,000
Deposits	190,000	93,000
Accrued Interest	7,000	4,000
Total	4,525,000	3,675,000
Consisting of		
Cash and Cash Equivalents—General Fund	1,150,000	400,000
Assets Whose Use Is Limited		
Corporate Funded Depreciation	1,950,000	1,800,000
Held by Trustee under Bond Indenture Agreements	1,425,000	1,475,000
Total	4,525,000	3,675,000

Note 3—Charity Care

The Hospital voluntarily provides free care to patients who lack financial resources and are deemed to be medically indigent. Such care is in compliance with the Hospital's mission. Because the Hospital does not pursue collection of amounts determined to qualify as charity care, they are not reported as revenue.

The Hospital maintains records to identify and monitor the level of charity care it provides. These records include the amount of charges forgone for services and supplies furnished under its charity care policy. During the years ended March 31, 20X8, and 20X7 such charges forgone totaled $395,000 and $375,000, respectively.

Note 4—Net Patient Service Revenue

The Hospital provides health care services through its inpatient and outpatient care facilities. The mix of receivables from patients and third-party payers at March 31, 20X8 and 20X7 is as follows:

	20X8	*20X7*
Medicare	30.0%	28.5%
Medicaid	15.0	16.0
Patients	13.0	12.5
Other third-party payers	42.0	43.0
Total	100.0%	100.0%

The Hospital has agreements with third-party payers that provide for payments to the Hospital at amounts different from its established rates. Contractual adjustments under third-party reimbursement programs represent the difference between the Hospital's established rates for services and amounts paid by third-party payers. A summary of the payment arrangements with major third-party payers follows:

Medicare. Inpatient acute care rendered to Medicare program beneficiaries is paid at prospectively determined rates-per-discharge. These rates vary according to a patient classification system that is based on clinical, diagnostic, and other factors. Inpatient nonacute care services and certain outpatient services are paid based upon either a cost reimbursement method, established fee screens, or a combination thereof. The Hospital is reimbursed for cost reimbursable items at a tentative rate with final settlement determination after submission of annual cost reports by the Hospital and audits by the Medicare fiscal intermediary. At the current year end, all Medicare settlements for the previous two years are subject to audit and retroactive adjustments.

Medicaid. Inpatient services rendered to Medicaid program beneficiaries are reimbursed at prospectively determined rates-per-day. Outpatient services rendered to Medicaid program beneficiaries are reimbursed at prospectively determined rates-per-visit.

Blue Cross. Inpatient services rendered to Blue Cross subscribers are reimbursed under a cost reimbursement methodology. The Hospital is reimbursed at a tentative rate with final settlement determined after submission of annual cost reports by the Hospital and audits by Blue Cross. The Blue Cross cost report for the prior year end is subject to audit and retroactive adjustment.

The Hospital has also entered into payment agreements with certain commercial insurance carriers, health maintenance organizations, and preferred provider organizations. The bases for payment under these agreements include discounts from established charges and prospectively determined daily rates.

Gross patient service revenue for services rendered by the Hospital under the Medicare, Medicaid, and Blue Cross payment agreements for the years ended March 31, 20X8 and 20X7 is approximately as follows:

	20X8		20X7	
	Amount	*%*	*Amount*	*%*
Medicare	$20,850,000	43.0	$19,900,000	42.0
Medicaid	10,190,000	21.0	10,200,000	21.5
All other payers	17,460,000	36.0	17,300,000	36.5
	$48,500,000	100.0	$47,400,000	100.0

Note 5—Property, Plant, and Equipment

The Hospital's property, plant, and equipment at March 31, 20X8 and 20X7 are as follows:

	20X8	20X7
Buildings and improvements	$14,700,000	$14,000,000
Land improvements	1,100,000	1,100,000
Equipment	28,900,000	27,600,000
Total	$44,700,000	$42,700,000
Accumulated depreciation	(26,100,000)	(24,200,000)
Net Depreciable Assets	$18,600,000	$18,500,000
Land	480,000	480,000
Construction in progress	220,000	220,000
Net Property, Plant, Equipment	$19,300,000	$19,200,000

Construction in progress, which involves a renovation project, has not progressed in the last twelve-month period because of a zoning dispute. The project will not require significant outlay to reach completion, as anticipated additional expenditures are currently estimated at $100,000.

Note 6—Long-Term Debt

Long-term debt consists of the following:

	20X8	20X7
Hospital Facility Revenue Bonds (Series 1995) at varying interest rates from 4.5% to 5.5%, depending on date of maturity through 2010.	$6,000,000	$6,500,000

The future maturities of long-term debt are as follows:

Years Ending March 31

20X7	$ 475,000
20X8	500,000
2XX0	525,000
2XX1	550,000
2XX2	575,000
2XX3	600,000
Thereafter	3,750,000

Under the terms of the Trust Indenture the following funds (held by the trustee) were established:

Interest Fund

The Hospital deposits (monthly) into the Interest Fund an amount equal to one-sixth of the next semi-annual interest payment due on the bonds.

Bond Sinking Fund

The Hospital deposits (monthly) into the Bond Sinking Fund an amount equal to one-twelfth of the principal due on the next July 1.

Debt Service Reserve Fund

The Debt Service Reserve Fund must be maintained at an amount equal to 10 percent of the aggregate principal amount of all bonds then outstanding. It is to be used to make up any deficiencies in the Interest Fund and Bond Sinking Fund.

Assets held by the trustee under the Trust Indenture at March 31, 20X8 and 20X7 are as follows:

	20X8	20X7
Interest Fund	$ 300,000	$ 325,000
Bond Sinking Fund	525,000	500,000
Debt Service Reserve	600,000	650,000
Total	$1,425,000	$1,475,000

Note 7—Commitments

At March 31, 20X8, the Hospital had commitments outstanding for a renovation project at the Hospital of approximately $100,000. Construction in progress on the renovation has not progressed in the last twelve-month period because of a zoning dispute. Upon resolution of the dispute, remaining construction costs will be funded from Corporate Funded Depreciation cash reserves.

SOLUTIONS TO PRACTICE EXERCISES

SOLUTION TO PRACTICE EXERCISE 5–I

	Intensive Care Unit	Laboratory	Laundry
Drugs requisitioned	X		
Pathology supplies		X	
Detergents and bleach			X
Nursing salaries	X		
Clerical salaries	X	X	X
Uniforms (for laundry aides)			X
Repairs (parts for microscopes)		X	

Note: If no clerical salaries are assigned to Laundry, this is an acceptable alternative solution.

SOLUTION TO PRACTICE EXERCISE 6–I

	Direct Cost	*Indirect Cost*
Managed care marketing expense	X	
Real estate taxes		X
Liability insurance		X
Clinic telephone expense	X	
Utilities (for the entire facility)		X
Emergency room medical supplies	X	

SOLUTION TO PRACTICE EXERCISE 6–II

In real life the solution to this exercise will depend upon factors unique to the particular organization. The following solution is a generic one.

	Responsibility Center	*Support Center*
Security	X	
Communications	X	
Ambulance services	X	
Medical records		X
Educational resources		X
Human resources		X

Reporting: Each Responsibility Center has a manager. All report to the Director.

SOLUTION TO PRACTICE EXERCISE 7–I

Step 1. Find the highest volume of 1,100 packs at a cost of $7,150 in September and the lowest volume of 100 packs at a cost of $1,010 in August.

Step 2. Compute the variable rate per pack as:

	# of Packs	*Training Pack Cost*
Highest volume	1,100	$7,150
Lowest volume	100	1,010
Difference	1,000	$6,140

Step 3. Divide the difference in cost ($6,140) by the difference in # of packs (1,000) to arrive at the variable cost rate:

$6,140 divided by 1,000 packs = $6.14 per pack

Step 4. Compute the fixed overhead rate as follows:

At the highest level:

Total cost	$7,150
Less: Variable portion?	
[1,100 packs × $6.14 @]	(6,754)
Fixed Portion of Cost	$ 396

At the lowest level:

Total cost	$1,010
Less: Variable portion	
[100 packs × $6.14 @]	(614)
Fixed Portion of Cost	$ 396

Proof totals: $396 fixed portion at both levels.

SOLUTION TO PRACTICE EXERCISE 7–II

Step 1. Divide costs into variable and fixed portions. In this case $3,450,000 times 40 percent equals $1,380,000 variable cost and $3,450,000 times 60 percent equals $2,070,000 fixed cost.

Step 2. Compute the contribution margin:

	Amount
Revenue	$3,500,000
Less variable cost	(1,380,000)
Contribution margin	$2,120,000
Less fixed cost	2,070,000
Operating income	$ 50,000

SOLUTION TO PRACTICE EXERCISE 7–III

	Amount	*%*	
Revenue	$1,210,000	100.00	
Less variable cost	(205,000)	16.94	
Contribution margin	$1,005,000	83.06	= PV or CM Ratio
Less fixed cost	(1,100,000)	90.91	
Operating loss	$(95,000)	7.85	

SOLUTION TO PRACTICE EXERCISE 8–I

1. *Compute Net Paid Days Worked*

Total days in business year		364
Less two days off per week		104
# Paid days per year		260
Less paid days not worked		
Holidays	8	
Sick days	5	
Education day	1	
Vacation days	5	
		19
Net paid days worked		241

2. *Convert Net Paid Days Worked to a Factor*

Total days in business year divided by net paid days worked equals factor

$$364/241 = 1.510373$$

SOLUTION TO PRACTICE EXERCISE 8–II

	Shift 1 Day	Shift 2 Evening	Shift 3 Night	=	24-Hour Scheduling Total
Position: Admissions officer	2	1	1		4 8-hour shifts
FTEs—to cover position					
7 days/week equals	2.8	1.4	1.4		5.6 FTEs
Position: Clerical	1	0	0		1 8-hour shift
FTEs—to cover position					
7 days/week equals	1.4	0	0		1.4 FTEs

SOLUTION TO PRACTICE EXERCISE 9–I

Current Liabilities	30,000
Total Assets	1,000,000
Income from Operations	80,000
Accumulated Depreciation	480,000
Total Operating Revenue	180,000
Current Portion of Long-Term Debt	10,000
Interest Income	-0-
Inventories	5,000

SOLUTION TO PRACTICE EXERCISE 9–II

1. Straight-line depreciation would amount to $54,000 per year for 10 years. This amount is computed as follows:

   Step 1. Compute the cost net of salvage or trade-in value: 600,000 less 10 percent salvage value or 60,000 equals 540,000.

   Step 2. Divide the resulting figure by the expected life (also known as estimated useful life): 540,000 divided by 10 equals 54,000 depreciation per year for 10 years.

2. Double declining depreciation is computed as follows:

   Step 1. Compute the straight-line rate: 1 divided by 10 equals 10 percent.

   Step 2. Now double the rate (as in "double declining method"): 10 percent times 2 equals 20 percent.

Step 3. Compute the first year's depreciation expense: 600,000 times 20 percent = 120,000.

Step 4. Compute the carry-forward book value at the beginning of the second year: 600,000 book value beginning Year 1 less Year 1 depreciation of 120,000 equals book value at beginning of the second year of 480,000.

Step 5. Compute the second year's depreciation expense: 480,000 times 20 percent = 96,000.

Step 6. Compute the carry-forward book value at the beginning of the third year: 480,000 book value beginning Year 2 less Year 2 depreciation of 96,000 equals book value at beginning of the third year of 384,000.

—Continue until the asset's salvage or trade-in value has been reached.

Book Value at Beginning of Year	Depreciation Expense	Book Value at End of Year
600,000	600,000 × 20% = 120,000	600,000 – 120,000 = 480,000
480,000	480,000 × 20% = 96,000	480,000 – 96,000 = 384,000
384,000	384,000 × 20% = 76,800	384,000 – 76,800 = 307,200
307,200	307,200 × 20% = 61,440	307,200 – 61,440 = 245,760
245,760	245,760 × 20% = 49,152	245,760 – 49,152 = 196,608
196,608	196,608 × 20% = 39,322	196,608 – 39,322 = 157,286
157,286	157,286 × 20% = 31,457	157,286 – 31,457 = 125,829
125,829	125,829 × 20% = 25,166	125,829 – 25,166 = 100,663
100,663	100,663 × 20% = 20,132	100,663 – 20,132 = 80,531
80,531	80,561 at 10th year:	80,561 – 20,561 = 60,000

—Balance remaining at end of tenth year represents the salvage or trade-in value.

Note: Under the double declining balance method, book value never reaches zero. Therefore, a company typically adopts the straight-line method at the point where straight line would exceed the double declining balance.

SOLUTION TO PRACTICE EXERCISE 10–I

Current Ratio

The current ratio is represented as Current Ratio = Current Assets divided by Current Liabilities. This ratio is considered to be a measure of short-term debt-paying ability. However, it must be carefully interpreted.

Current Ratio Computation

$$\frac{\text{Current Assets}}{\text{Current Liabilities}} = \frac{\$70,000}{\$30,000} = 2.33 \text{ to } 1$$

Quick Ratio

The quick ratio is represented as Quick Ratio = Cash + Short-Term Investments + Net Receivables divided by Current Liabilities. This ratio is considered to be an even more severe test of short-term debt-paying ability (even more severe than the current ratio). The quick ratio is also known as the acid-test ratio, for obvious reasons.

$$\frac{\text{Cash \& Cash Equivalents} + \text{Net Receivables}}{\text{Current Liabilities}} = \frac{\$65,000}{\$30,000} = 2.167 \text{ to } 1$$

SOLUTION TO PRACTICE EXERCISE 10–II

Solvency Ratios

Debt Service Coverage Ratio (DSCR)

The Debt Service Coverage Ratio (DSCR) is represented as change in unrestricted net assets (net income) plus interest, depreciation, and amortization divided by maximum annual debt service. This ratio is universally used in credit analysis, and figures prominently in the Mini-Case Study #1.

$$\frac{\substack{\text{Change in Unrestricted Net Assets (net income)} \\ \text{plus Interest, Depreciation, Amortization}}}{\text{Maximum Annual Debt Service}} = \frac{\$113,100}{\$22,200} = 5.1$$

Note: $80,000 + $3,100 + $30,000 = $113,100.

Liabilities To Fund Balance (or Debt to Net Worth)

The liabilities to fund balance or net worth computation is represented as total liabilities divided by unrestricted net assets (fund balances) (or net worth) = total debt divided by tangible net worth. This figure is a quick indicator of debt load.

$$\frac{\text{Total Liabilities}}{\text{Unrestricted Fund Balance}} = \frac{\$200,000}{\$800,000} = 2.5$$

SOLUTION TO PRACTICE EXERCISE 10–III

Profitability Ratios

Operating Margin

The operating margin, which is generally expressed as a percentage, is represented as operating income (loss) divided by total operating revenues. This ratio is used for a number of managerial purposes and also sometimes enters into credit analysis. It is therefore a multi-purpose measure.

$$\frac{\text{Operating Income (Loss)}}{\text{Total Operating Revenues}} = \frac{\$80,000}{\$180,000} = 44.4\%$$

Return on Total Assets

The return on total assets is represented as earnings before interest and taxes (EBIT) divided by total assets. This is a broad measure in common use.

$$\frac{\text{EBIT (Earnings Before Interest \& Taxes)}}{\text{Total Assets}} = \frac{\$83,100}{\$1,000,000} = 8.3\%$$

Note: $80,000 + $3,100 = $83,100

SOLUTION TO PRACTICE EXERCISE 11–I: UNADJUSTED RATE OF RETURN

1. Calculation using original investment amount:

$$\frac{\$100,000}{\$500,000} = 20\% \text{ Unadjusted Rate of Return}$$

2. Calculation using average investment amount:

   First Step: Compute average investment amount for total unrecovered asset cost:

At beginning of estimated useful life	= $500,000
At end of estimated useful life	= $ 50,000
Sum	$550,000

   Divided by 2 = $275,000 average investment amount

   Second Step: Calculate unadjusted rate of return:

$$\frac{\$100,000}{\$275,000} = 36.4\% \text{ Unadjusted Rate of Return}$$

SOLUTION TO PRACTICE EXERCISE 11–II: FINDING THE FUTURE VALUE (WITH A COMPOUND INTEREST TABLE)

Step 1. Refer to the Compound Interest Table found in Appendix 11–B at the back of this chapter. Reading across, or horizontally, find the 7 percent column. Reading down, or vertically, find Year 6. Trace across the Year 6 line item to the 7 percent column. The factor is 1.501.

Step 2. Multiply the current savings account balance of $11,000 times the factor of 1.501 to find the future value of $16,511. In six years at compound interest of 7 percent, the college fund will have a balance of $16,511.

SOLUTION TO PRACTICE EXERCISE 11–III:
FINDING THE PRESENT VALUE

Step 1. Refer to the Present Value Table found in Appendix 11–A at the back of this chapter. Reading across, or horizontally, find the 7 percent column. Reading down, or vertically, find Year 15. Trace across the Year 15 line item to the 7 percent column. The factor is 0.3624.

Step 2. Multiply $150,000 times the factor of 0.3624 to find the present value of $54,360.

SOLUTION TO PRACTICE EXERCISE 11–IV

Assemble the assumptions in an orderly manner:

Assumption 1: Initial cost of the investment = $16,950.
Assumption 2: Estimated annual net cash inflow the investment will generate = $3,000.
Assumption 3: Useful life of the asset = 10 years.

Perform calculation:

Step 1: Divide the initial cost of the investment ($16,950) by the estimated annual net cash inflow it will generate ($3,000). The answer is a ratio amounting to 5.650.

Step 2: Now use the abbreviated look-up table for the Present Value of an Annuity of $1, which is found at the back of the Examples and Exercises section. Find the line item for the number of periods that matches the useful life of the asset (10 years in this case).

Step 3: Look across the 10 year line on the table and find the column that approximates the ratio of 5.650 (as computed in Step 1). That column contains the interest rate representing the rate of return. In this case the rate of return is 12 percent.

SOLUTION TO PRACTICE EXERCISE 11–V

Assemble assumptions in an orderly manner:

Assumption 1: Purchase price of the equipment = $500,000.
Assumption 2: Useful life of the equipment = 10 years.
Assumption 3: Revenue the machine will generate per year = $84,000.
Assumption 4: Direct operating costs associated with earning the revenue = $21,000.
Assumption 5: Depreciation expense per year (computed as purchase price per assumption 1 divided by useful life per assumption 2) = $50,000.

Perform computation:

Step 1: Find the machine's expected net income after taxes:

Revenue (Assumption 3)	$84,000
Less	
Direct operating costs (Assumption 4)	$21,000
Depreciation (Assumption 5)	50,000
	71,000
Net income	$13,000

Note: No income taxes for this hospital.

Step 2: Find the net annual cash inflow the machine is expected to generate (in other words, convert the net income to a cash basis).

Net income	$13,000
Add back depreciation (a noncash expenditure)	50,000
Annual net cash inflow after taxes	$63,000

Step 3: Compute the payback period:

$$\frac{\text{Investment}}{\text{Net annual cash inflow}} = \frac{\$500,000 \text{ machine cost*}}{\$63,000} = 7.9 \text{ year payback period}$$

*assumption 1 above
**per Step 2 above

The machine will pay back its investment under these assumptions in 7% years.

SOLUTION TO PRACTICE EXERCISE 12–I

Common sizing for the assets of the two hospitals appears on the worksheet below. Note that their gross numbers are very different, yet the proportionate relationships of the percentages (20 percent, 75 percent, and 5 percent) are the same for both hospitals.

	Same Year for Both Hospitals			
	Hospital A		*Hospital B*	
Current assets	$ 2,000,000	20%	$ 8,000,000	20%
Property, plant, and equipment	7,500,000	75%	30,000,000	75%
Other assets	500,000	5%	2,000,000	5%
Total assets	$10,000,000	100%	$40,000,000	100%

Solution to Practice Exercise 12–II

	Year 1	*Year 2*	*Difference*	
		Hospital A		
Current assets	$1,600,000	$ 2,000,000	$ 400,000	25%
Property, plant, and equipment	6,000,000	7,500,000	1,500,000	25%
Other assets	400,000	500,000	100,000	25%
Total assets	$8,000,000	$10,000,000	$2,000,000	—

Note: The worksheet below shows Hospital A with both common sizing and trend analysis:

	Year 1		*Year 2*		*Difference*	
			Hospital A			
Current assets	$1,600,000	20%	$ 2,000,000	20%	$ 400,000	25%
Property, plant, and equipment	6,000,000	75%	7,500,000	75%	1,500,000	25%
Other assets	400,000	5%	500,000	5%	100,000	25%
Total assets	$8,000,000	100%	$10,000,000	100%	$2,000,000	—

SOLUTION TO PRACTICE EXERCISE 13–I

Your initial budget assumptions were as follows:

Assume the budget anticipated 30,000 inpatient days this year at an average of $650 revenue per day, or $19,500,000. Further assume that inpatient expenses were budgeted at $600 per patient day, or $18,000,000. Also assume the budget anticipated 10,000 outpatient visits this year at an average of $400 revenue per visit, or $4,000,000. Further assume that outpatient expenses were budgeted at $380 per visit, or $3,800,000. The budget worksheet would look like this:

	As Budgeted
Revenue—Inpatient	$19,500,000
Revenue—Outpatient	4,000,000
Subtotal	$23,500,000
Expenses—Inpatient	$18,000,000
Expenses—Outpatient	3,800,000
Subtotal	$21,800,000
Excess of revenue over expenses	$1,700,000

Now assume that only 27,000, or 90 percent, of the patient days are going to actually be achieved for the year. The average revenue of $650 per day will be achieved for these 27,000 days (thus 27,000 times 650 equals 17,550,000). Also assume that outpatient visits will actually amount to 110 percent, or 11,000 for the year. The average revenue of $400 per visit will be achieved for these 11,000 visits (thus 11,000 times 400 equals 4,400,000). Further assume that, due to the heroic efforts of the Chief Financial Officer, the actual inpatient expenses will amount to $11,600,000 and the actual outpatient expenses will amount to $4,000,000. The actual results would look like this:

	Actual
Revenue—Inpatient	$17,550,000
Revenue—Outpatient	4,400,000
Subtotal	$21,950,000
Expenses—Inpatient	16,100,000
Expenses—Outpatient	4,000,000
Subtotal	$20,100,000
Excess of revenue over expenses	$1,850,000

Since the budgeted revenues and expenses still reflect the original expectations of 30,000 inpatient days and 10,000 outpatient visits, the budget report would look like this:

	Actual	*Budget*	*Static Budget Variance*
Revenue—Inpatient	$17,550,000	$19,500,000	$(1,950,000)
Revenue—Outpatient	4,400,000	4,000,000	400,000
Subtotal	$21,950,000	$23,500,000	$(1,550,000)
Expenses—Inpatient	$16,100,000	$18,000,000	$(1,900,000)
Expenses—Outpatient	4,000,000	3,800,000	200,000
Subtotal	$20,100,000	$21,800,000	$(1,700,000)
Excess of revenue over expenses	$ 1,850,000	$ 1,700,000	$ 150,000

Note: The negative effect of the $1,550,000 net drop in revenue is offset by the greater effect of the $1,700,000 net drop in expenses, resulting in a positive net effect of $150,000.

REQUIRED SOLUTION TO PRACTICE EXERCISE 13–II

The Price Variance is $206,100 (3,435,000 less 3,228,900 equals 206,100).
The Quantity Variance is $185,000 (3,435,000 less 3,250,000 equals 185,000).

OPTIONAL SOLUTION TO PRACTICE EXERCISE 13–II

The $3,228,900 actual overhead costs represent 687,000 RVUs times $4.70 per RVU.
The $3,250,000 budgeted overhead costs represent 650,000 RVUs times $5.00 per RVU.

Index

About the Authors

Judith J. Baker, PhD, CPA, is Executive Director of Resource Group, Ltd., a Dallas-based health care consulting firm. She earned her Bachelor of Science degree in Business Administration at the University of Missouri, Columbia and her Master of Liberal Studies with a concentration in Business Management at the University of Oklahoma, Norman. She earned her Master of Arts and Doctorate in Human and Organizational Systems, with a concentration in costing systems, at the Fielding Institute, Santa Barbara, California. She is an adjunct faculty member at the Case Western Reserve University Frances Payne Bolton School of Nursing.

Judith has over thirty years experience in health care and consults on numerous health care systems and costing problems. She has worked with health care systems, costing, and reimbursement throughout her career. As a HCFA subcontractor she assists in validation of costs for new programs and for rate setting and consults on cost report design.

Note: Needs to be edited by author:

Judith has written over 40 articles, manuals, and books. She is Consulting Editor for Aspen Publishers, Inc. Her latest books are Activity-Based Costing and Activity-Based Management for Health Care, Prospective Payment for Long-Term Care: An Annual Guide, and Prospective Payment for Home Health Agencies (all Aspen publications). She is co-editor of the quarterly Journal of Healthcare Finance.

R.W. Baker, JD, is Managing Partner of Resource Group, Ltd., a Dallas-based health care consulting firm. He has more than 30 years of experience in health care and has designed, directed, and administered numerous financial impact studies for health care providers. His recent studies have centered around facility-specific MDS data collection and analysis. He and his firm have subcontracted to the HCFA Nursing Home Case Mix and Quality Demonstration from 1990 to present.

Note: Needs to be edited by author:

R.W. is the editor of continuing professional education seminar manuals and training manuals for facility personnel and for research staff members. He is a Consulting Editor with Aspen Publishers, Inc. and is co-author of A Step-by-Step Guide to the Minimum Data Set (Aspen Publishers, Inc. 1999).